Contents

Section III RECOGNITION AND TREATMENT OF TRAVEL-RELATED ILLNESS

Section IV TRAVEL-RELATED INFECTIOUS DISEASES AND OTHER AILMENTS

Contributors

Nathaniel James, MD
Director, International Clinic
Maine Medical Center
Portland, Maine

Carol McCarthy, MD
Chief, Pediatric Infectious Disease
Maine Medical Center
Portland, Maine

Devayani Namassivaya, MD
Infectious Disease Specialist
Erie County Medical Center
Buffalo, New York

Stephen D. Sears, MD, MPH
Senior Vice President for Medical Administration
MaineGeneral Medical Center, Augusta, Maine
Adjunct Associate Professor, Family and Community Medicine
Dartmouth Medical School, Hanover, New Hampshire

Robert P. Smith, MD, MPH
Clinical Professor of Medicine
University of Vermont School of Medicine
Burlington, Vermont
Division of Infectious Disease
Maine Medical Center, Portland, Maine

Preface

The explosive growth in international travel and the increasing popularity of adventurous travel itineraries create new challenges for primary care providers. Nearly 50 million travelers from industrialized countries visit developing countries each year, and many of them rely on their family physicians for initial advice on medical preparation for their trip. Although specialized "travel clinics" flourish to meet this need in many urban areas, many travelers either do not have access to these services or prefer to see their family doctor first. In addition, as travelers seek ever more remote areas, and as "expedition" type travel becomes common, returning travelers with illness seek help from their regular physicians, who may refer them to any of several specialists (in infectious disease, gastroenterology, neurology, dermatology, etc.), depending on the nature of their ailment. Frequently, the fact of their travel introduces diagnostic considerations that are not routine for most physicians practicing in developed countries.

It is the purpose of this book to serve as a ready reference for medical providers as they prepare travelers for their trip and as they evaluate travelers on their return. This book is not intended to be comprehensive, but rather a starting point for the clinician encountering the fascinating challenges of "travel medicine." It should be used in conjunction with the CDC's annually updated and excellent publication, *Health Information for International Travel*. The CDC provides on-line and hot-line information as well, as do several excellent resources listed in Appendix 3.

The first two sections of this book are designed to provide a summary of key issues in the provision of pretravel advice, including the use of required and recommended vaccines, options for prevention of malaria and when to consider them, the preparation of travelers for encounters with the common ailment of traveler's diarrhea, and preparing for the new challenges implicit in the exploration of new environments. Special considerations are included for travelers with chronic diseases, such as diabetes and HIV, as well as for pregnant women and for children.

The third section of this book is designed to aid in the initial evaluation of returning travelers. In addition to an approach to screening asymptomatic travelers and immigrants, it includes chapters devoted to common disease syndromes, such as fever, gastroenteritis, dermatitis, or eosinophilia.

The final section of the book includes detailed information on specific diseases. It is hoped that reference to this section will help to broaden the differential diagnosis of common complaints. The focus here is on diseases often linked to travel rather than on cosmopolitan diseases that are always in the differential diagnosis. Whereas a few very rare diseases are included, an effort has been made to designate them as such. The purpose is not to stimulate the pursuit of zebras at the first sound of hoof beats, but to heighten awareness of the geographic differences in disease occurrence.

At the end of the book are three Appendixes. Appendix 1 is a list of diseases by geography, as prepared by the CDC. Appendix 2 is a list of antiparasitic drugs. Appendix 3 lists a number of excellent resources, both electronic and printed, that can provide information of greater depth and breadth for the interested physician.

Although this book is prepared with the North American physician in mind, we recognize that the impact of most of the diseases discussed is minimal by that reference point compared to their impact in endemic areas. It is our hope that the growth of travel medicine will stimulate increasing interest in the global impact of these diseases, and that the resources to curb these diseases where they are most morbid will be vigorously pursued.

Robert P. Smith, MD
Stephen D. Sears, MD

Acknowledgments

This handbook benefits from the availability of an increasing array of superb resources on travel medicine. For the preparation of travelers, excellent and comprehensive texts include Dupont and Steffen's *Textbook of Travel Medicine and Health*, their succinct *Manual of Travel Medicine and Health*, and *The Travel and Tropical Medicine Manual* by Jong and McMullen. A section of the CDC's *Health Information for International Travel* is included in our Appendix 1, as are several tables and maps in the text.

For preparation of disease-oriented information, we have relied on the template created by Drs. Onion and Sears for Blackwell's Primary Care Essentials Series. Some of these sections have been "globalized" to focus more on disease geography, risk to travelers, and prevention. Many additional disease outlines have been added to cover the array of considerations commonly encompassed by travel and tropical medicine. In this effort, two texts have proven extraordinarily helpful. Wilson's *A World Guide to Infections* remains a unique and invaluable resource, and we have relied in some instances on this reference for information on disease risk. Guerrant's two-volume *Tropical Infectious Diseases* provided us with a superb and comprehensive reference for updated disease specific information. In addition, the "Travel Medicine" issue (1998) of the *Infectious Disease Clinics of North America* has been another excellent resource.

Drs. Nathaniel James and Carol McCarthy of Maine Medical Center contributed sections on health screening for immigrants and on travel with children, and Dr. Devayani Namassivaya contributed to sections on the treatment of malaria, filariasis, giardiasis, and typhoid fever. We also want to thank our travel clinic nurses—Doris Zappala, Karla Gottstine, and Carole Duperre—who have increased our awareness of the nuances of travel medicine. Finally, we would like to thank Dan Onion, MD, originator and editor of the Primary Care Essentials Series, and Julia Casson and Chris Davis of Blackwell Science, for their assistance and patience.

Notice

The indications and dosages of all drugs in this book have been recommended in the medical literature and conform to the practices of the general community. The medications described and treatment prescriptions suggested do not necessarily have specific approval by the Food and Drug Administration for use in the diseases and dosages for which they are recommended. The package insert for each drug should be consulted for use and dosage as approved by the FDA. Because standards for usage change, it is advisable to keep abreast of revised recommendations, particularly those concerning new drugs.

Medical Abbreviations

A_2	Aortic (first) component of S_2
ab	Antibodies
ABGs	Arterial blood gases
ac	Before meals
ACE	Angiotensin convertine enzyme
ACEI	ACE imhibitor
Ach	Acetylcholine
ACLS	Advanced cardiac life support
ACOG	American College of Obstetrics and Gynecology
ACTH	Adrenocorticotropic hormone
AD	Right ear
ADH	Antidiuretic hormone
ADHD	Attention deficit hyperactivity disorder
ADLs	Activities of daily living
AF	Atrial fibrillation
AFB	Acid-fast bacillus
Afib	Atrial fibrillation
AFP	Alpha fetoprotein
Aflut	Atrial flutter
ag	Antigen
AGN	Acute glomerular nephritis
AI	Aortic insufficiency
aka	Also known as
Al	Aluminum
ALA	α levulinic acid
ALS	Amyotrophic lateral sclerosis
ALL	Acute lymphocytic leukemia
ALT	SGPT; alanine transferase
AMI	Anterior myocardial infarction
AMS	Acute mountain sickness
ANA	Antinuclear antibody

ANCA	Antineutrophil cytoplasmic autoantibodies
AODM	Adult onset diabetes mellitus
AP	Anterior-posterior
AR	Aldose reductase
ARA	Angiotensin receptor antagonist
ARDS	Adult respiratory distress syndrome
AS	Aortic stenosis, or left ear
ASA	Aspirin
ASCVD	Arteriosclerotic cardiovascular disease
ASD	Atrial septal defect
ASHD	Arteriosclerotic heart disease
ASLO	Antistreptolysin O titer
ASO	Antistreptolysin O titer
AST	SGOT; aspartate transferase
asx	Asymptomatic
atm	Atmospheres
ATN	Acute tubular necrosis
AU	Both ears
AV	Arteriovenous; or atrial-ventricular
AVM	Ateriovenous malformation
Ba	Barium
bact	Bacteriology
BAL	British anti-Lewisite
BCG	Bacille Calmette-Guérin
BCLS	Basic cardiac life support
BE	Barium enema
bid	twice a day
BiPAP	Bi (2)-positive airway pressures
biw	twice a week
BJ	Bence Jones
bm	bowel movement
BM	Basement membrane
BP	Blood pressure
BPH	Benign prostatic hypertrophy
BS	Blood sugar
BSE	Breast self-exam
BSOO	Bilateral salpingo-oophorectomy
BUN	Blood urea nitrogen
bx	Biopsy

C′	Complement
Ca	Calcium, or cancer depending on context
CABG	Coronary artery bypass graft
CAD	Coronary artery disease
cAMP	Cyclic AMP
cath	Catheterization
CBC	Complete blood count
cc	Cubic centimeter
CEA	Carcinoembryonic antigen
cf	Compare
CF	Complement fixation antibodies
CHD	Congenital heart disease
chem	Chemistries
chemoRx	Chemotherapy
CHF	Congestive heart failure
CI	Cardiac index
CIN	Cervical intraepithelial neoplasia
CIS	Carcinoma in situ
Cl	Chloride
CLL	Chronic lymphocytic leukemia
CMF	Cytoxan, methotrexate, 5-FU
CML	Chronic myelocytic leukemia
cmplc	Complications
CMV	Cystomegalovirus
CN	Cranial nerve; or cyanide
CNS	Central nervous system
CO	Cardiac output
c/o	Complaining of
col	Colonies
COPD	Chronic obstructive lung disease
cp	Cerebellar-pontine
CP	Cerebral palsy
CPAP	Continuous positive airway pressure
CPC	Clinical/pathologic conference
CPG	Coproporphyrinogen
CPK	Creatine phophokinase
CPR	Cardiopulmonary resuscitation
cps	Cycles per second
CREST	Calcinosis, Raynaud's, esophageal reflux, sclerodactyly, telangiectasias

CRH	Corticotropin releasing hormone.
crit	Hematocrit
CRP	C reactive protein
crs	Course
c + s	Culture and sensitivity
C/S	Cesarian section
CSF	Cerebrospinal fluid
CT	Computerized tomography
Cu	Copper
CVA	Cerebrovascular accident
CVP	Central venous pressure
d	Day(s)
dB	Decibel
DAT	Dementia, Alzheimer's type
DBCT	Double blind controlled trial
DCS	Decompression sickness
DHS	Delayed hypersensitivity
DI	Diabetes insipidus
dias	Diastolic
DIC	Disseminated intravascular coagulation
dig	Digoxin
dip	Distal interphalangeal joint
DJD	Degenerative joint disease
DKA	Diabetic ketoacidosis
DMSA	Dimercaptosuccinic acid
DNA	Deoxyribonucleic acid
d/o	Disorder
DOE	Dyspnea on exertion
DPG	Diphosphoglycerate
DPN	Diphosphopyridine nucleotide
DPNH	Reduced DPN
DPT	Diphtheria, pertussis, tetanus vaccine
DS	Double strength
dT	Diphtheria tetanus adult vaccine
DTRs	Deep tendon reflexes
DTs	Delerium tremens
DU	Duodenal ulcer
DVT	Deep venous thrombosis
dx	Diagnosis or diagnostic

EACA	ε-aminocaproic acid
EBV	Ebstein-Barr virus
ECM	Erythema chronicum marginatum
EF	Ejection fraction
EGD	Esophagogastroduodenoscopy
ELISA	Enzyme-linked immunosorbent assay
E/M	Erythroid/myeloid
EM	Electron microscopy
EMG	Electromyogram
esp	Especially
Endo	Endoscopy
Epidem	Epidemiology
ER	Estrogen receptors; or emergency room
ERCP	Endoscopic retrograde cholangio-pancreatography
ERT	Estrogen replacement therapy
ESR	Erythrocyte sedimentation rate
et	Endotracheal
ETOH	Ethanol
ETT	Exercise tolerance test

F	Female; or Fahrenheit
FA	Fluorescent antibody, or folic acid
FBS	Fasting blood sugar
Fe	Iron
FFA	Free fatty acids
FIGLU	Formiminoglutamic acid
fl	Femtoliter
FMF	Familial Mediterrranean fever
FSH	Follicle stimulating hormone
FTA	Fluorescent treponemal antibody
FTT	Failure to thrive
f/u	Follow up
FUO	Fever of unknown origin
FVC	Forced vital capacity
fx	Fracture

g	Gauge
GABA	γ-Aminobutyric acid
gc	Gonorrhea
GE	Gastroesophageal

GFR	Glomerular filtration rate
GHRH	Growth hormone releasing hormone
gi	Gastrointestinal
glu	glucose
glut	Glutamine
gm	Gram
GN	Glomerulonephritis
GnRH	Gonadotropin releasing hormone
GTT	Glucose tolerance test
gtts	Drops
gu	Genitourinary
GVHD	Graft vs. host disease
HACE	High altitude cerebral edema
HAPE	High altitude pulmonary edema
HBIG	Hepatitis B immune globulin
HCl	Hydrochloric acid
HCO_3	Bicarbonate
hct	Hematocrit
HDL	High density lipoprotein
H & E	Hematoxylin and eosin
hem	Hematology
hep	Hepatitis
H. flu	Hemophilus influenza
Hg	Mercury
hgb	Hemoglobin
$HgbA_1C$	Hemoglobin A_1C level
HGH	Human growth hormone
5-HIAA	5-Hydroxy indole acedic acid
Hib	Hemophilus influenza B vaccine
his	Histidine
HIV	Human immunodeficiency virus
HLA	Human leukocyte antigens
HMG-COA	Hydroxymethylglutaryl-coenzyme A
h/o	History of
H + P	History and physical
hpf	High power field
HPV	Human papilloma virus
hr	Hour(s)

HRIG	Human rabies immune globulin
hs	At bedtime
HSP	Henoch-Schonlein purpura
HSV	Herpes simplex virus
HT	Hypertension
5HT	5-Hydroxytryptophan
HUS	Hemolytic uremic syndrome
HVA	Homovanillic acid
hx	History
I or I_2	Iodine
IADLs	Instumental activities of daily living
IBD	Inflammatory bowel disease
ICU	Intensive care unit
I + D	Incision and drainage
IDDM	Insulin dependent diabetes melitus
IEP	Immunoelectrophoresis
IF	Intrinsic factor
IFA	Immunofluorescent antibody
IgA	Immunoglobulin A
IgE	Immunoglobulin E
IgG	Immunoglobulin G
IgM	Immunoglobulin M
IHSS	Idiopathic hypertrophicsubaortic stenosis
im	Intramuscular
incr	Increased
INH	Isoniazid
INR	International normalized ratio
IP	Interphalangeal
IPG	Impedance plethysmography
IPPB	Intermittent positive pressure breathing
IPPD	Intermediate purified protein derivative
ITP	Idiopathic thrombocytopenic purpura
IU	International units
IUD	Intrauterine device
IUGR	Intrauterine growth retardation
IVC	Inferior vena cava
IVP	Intravenous pyelogram
IWMI	Inferior wall myocardial infarction

J	Joule
JODM	Juvenile onset diabetes mellitus
JRA	Juvenile rheumatoid arthritis
JVD	Jugular venous distension
JVP	Jugular venous pressure/pulse
K	Potassium
kg	Kilogram
KOH	Potassium hydroxide
KS	Kaposi's sarcoma
KUB	Abdominal xray ("kidneys, ureters, bladder")
L	Liter; or left
LA	Left atrium; or long acting if after a drug
LAP	Leukocyte alkaline phosphatase
LATS	Long acting thyroid stimulating protein
LBBB	Left bundle branch block
LDH	Lactate dehydrogenase
LDL	Low density lipoproteins
LES	Lower esophageal sphincter
LFTs	Liver function tests
LH	Luteinizing hormone
LHRH	LH releasing hormone
LMW	Low molecular weight
LP	Lumbar puncture
LS	Lumbosacral
LV	Left ventricle
LVH	Left ventricular hypertrophy
lytes	Electrolytes
m	Meter(s)
M	Male
MAI	Mycobacterium avium intracellulare
MAO	Monamine oxidase
mcp	Metacarpal-phalangeal joint(s)
MD	Muscular dystrophy; or physician
MDI	Metered dose inhaler
meds	Medications
MEN	Multiple endocrine neoplasias
mEq	Millieqivalent

mets	Metastases
METS	Metabolic equivalents
mg	Milligram
Mg	Magnesium
MHC	Major histocompatibility locus
MI	Myocardial infarction/ or mitral insufficiency
MIC	Minimum inhibitory concentration
min	Minute
MMR	Measles, mumps, rubella
mOsm	Milliosmole/s
mp	Metocarpal phalangeal
6MP	6-mercaptopurine
MR	Mitral regurgitation
MRA	Magnetic resonance angiography
MRFIT	Multiple risk factor intervention trial
MRI	Magnetic resonance imaging
MRSA	Methicillin resistant staph aureus
MS	Multiple sclerosis; or mitral stenosis
MSH	Melanocyte stimulating hormone
mtx	Methotrexate
Multip	Multiparous pt
μ	Micron
μgm	Microgram
Na	Sodium
NAD	Nicotinamide adenine dinucleotide
NADH	Reduced form of NAD
NCI	National Cancer Institute
ncnc	normochromic normocytic
NCV	Nerve conduction velocities
neb	nebulizer
neg	negative
NG	Nasogastric
NH_3	Ammonia
NICU	Newborn intensive care unit
NIDDM	Noninsulin-dependent diabetes mellitus
nl	Normal
nL	Nanoliter
nm	Nanometer
NMRI	Nuclear magnetic resonance imaging

NNH	Number needed to harm
NNT	Number needed to treat
noninv	Noninvasive laboratory
NPH	Normal pressure hydrocephalus
npo	Nothing by mouth
NS	Normal saline
NSAID	Nonsteroidal anti-inflammatory drug
NSR	Normal sinus rythmn
NST	Nonstress test
Nullip	Nulliparous pt
NV + D	Nausea, vomiting and diarrhea

O_2	Oxygen
OB	Obstetrics
OCD	Obsessive compulsive disorder
OD	Overdose; or right eye
OGTT	Oral glucose tolerance test
OH	Hydroxy-
OM	Otitis media
op	Operative, or outpatient
O + P	Ova and parasites
OPD	Outpatient department
OPV	Oral polio vaccine
OS	Left eye
osm	Osmoles
OTC	Over the counter
OU	Both eyes
oz	Ounce

P	Pulse
P_2	Pulmonary (2nd) component of S_2
PA	Pernicious anemia; or pulmonary artery
PABA	Paraminobenzoic acid
PAC	Premature atrial contraction
PAF	Paroxysmal atrial fibrillation
PAN	Polyarteritis nodosa
Pap	Papanicolaou
PAP	Pulmonary artery pressure
par	Parenteral
PAS	p-Amino salicylic acid

PAT	Paroxysmal atrial tachycardia
Pathophys	Pathophysiology
Pb	Lead
PBG	Porphobilinogen
pc	After meals
PCP	Pneumocystis pneumonia
PCTA	Percutaneous transluminal angioplasty
PCR	Polymerase chain reaction
PCWP	Pulmonary capillary wedge pressure
PDA	Patent ductus arteriosus
PEG	Percutaneous endoscopic gastrostomy
PEP	Protein electrophoresis
PFTs	Pulmonary function tests
PG	Prostaglandin
phos	Phosphatase
PI	Pulmonic insufficiency
PID	Pelvic inflammatory disease
PIH	Pregnancy induced hypertension
pip	Proximal interphalangeal joint
PMI	Point of maximal impulse of heart
PMNLs	Polymorphonuclear leukocytes
PMR	Polymyalgia rheumatica
PND	Paroxysmal nocturnal dyspnea
PNH	Paroxysmal hemoglobinuria
po	By mouth
PO_4	Phosphate
polys	Polymorphonuclear leukocytes
POPS	Pulmonary overpressurization syndrome
pos	Positive
PP	Protoporphyrin
ppd	Pack per day
PPD	Tuberculin skin test
PPG	Protoporphyrinogen
pr	By rectum
pRBBB	Partial right bundle branch block
pre-op	Pre-operative
prep	Preparation
primip	Primiparous pt
prn	As needed
PROM	Premature rupture of membranes

PS	Pulmonic stenosis
PSA	Prostate specific antigen
PSVT	Paroxysmal supraventricular tachycardia
PT	Protime
pt(s)	Patient(s)
PTH	Parathormone
PTT	Partial thromboplastin time
PUD	Peptic ulcer disease
PUVA	Psoralen + UVA light
PVC	Premature ventricular tachycardia
q	Every
qd	Daily
qid	4 times a day
qod	Every other day
qow	Every other week
qt	Quart
R	Right, or respirations
RA	Rheumatoid arthritis
RAIU	Radioactive iodine uptake
RAST	Radioallergosorbent test
RBBB	Right bundle branch block
rbc	Red blood cell
RCT	Randomized controlled trial
RDS	Respiratory distress syndrome
re	About
REM	Rapid eye movement
RES	Reticuloendothelial system
retic	Reticulocyte/s
Rh	Rhesus factor
RHD	Rheumatic heart disease
RIA	Radioimmunoassay
RIBA	Radio-immuno blot assay
RMSF	Rocky mountain spotted fever
ROM	Range of motion
ROS	Review of systems
RNA	Ribonucleic acid
RNP	Ribonucleoprotein
r/o	Rule out

RSV	Respiratory syncytial virus
RTA	Renal tubular acidosis
rv	Review
RV	Right ventricle
RVH	Right ventricular hypertrophy
rx	Treatment
S_1	First heart sound
S_2	Second heart sound
S_3	Third heart sound, gallop
S_4	Fourth heart sound, gallop
SAB	Spontaneous abortion
SAH	Subarachnoid hemorrhage
Sb	Antimony
SBE	Subacute bacterial endocarditis
sc	Subcutaneous
SD	Standard deviation
sens	Sensitivity
SER	Smooth endoplasmic reticulum
serol	Serology(ies)
SGA	Small for gestational age
si	Signs
SI	Sacroiliac
SIADH	Syndrome of inappropriate ADH
SIDS	Sudden infant death syndrome
SKSD	Streptokinase, streptodornase
sl	Sublingual
SLE	Systemic lupus erythematosis
SNF	Skilled nursing facility
soln	Solution
s/p	Status post
specif	Specificity
SPEP	Serum protein electrophoresis
SR	Slow release
SRS	Slow reacting substance
SS	Sickle cell disease
SSKI	Saturated solution of potassium iodide
SSRI	Selective serotonin reuptake inhibitor
SSS	Sick sinus syndrome
Staph	Staphylococcus

STD	Sexually transmitted disease
STS	Serologic test for syphilis
SVC	Superior vena cava
SVT	Supraventricular tachycardia
sx	Symptom(s)
sys	Systolic
T°	Fever/temperature
T_3	Triiodothyronine
T_4	Thyroxin
TA	Temporal arteritis
T + A	Tonsillectomy and adenoidectomy
tab	Tablet
TAH	Total abdominal hysterectomy
tbc	Tuberculosis
TCAs	Tricyclic antidepressants
TBG	Thyroid binding globulin
tcn	Tetracycline
Td	Tetanus/diphtheria, adult type
TD	Traveler's diarrhea
TEE	Transesophageal echocardiogram
TENS	Transcutaneious electrical nerve stimulation
Tfx	Transfusion
TI	Tricuspid insufficiency
TIA	Transient ischemic attack
TIBC	Total iron binding capacity
tid	3 times a day
TIPS	Transjugular intrahepatic porto-systemic shunt
tiw	Three times a week
TM	Tympanic membrane
Tm	Trimethoprim
Tm/S	Trimethoprim/sulfa
TNF	Tumor necrosis factor
TNG	Nitroglycerine
TPA	Tissue plasminogen activator
TPN	Total parental nutrition
TPNH	Triphosphopyridine reduced
TRH	Thyroid releasing hormone
TS	Tricuspid stenosis

TSH	Thyroid stimulating hormone
TTP	Thrombotic thrombocytopenic purpura
TURP	Transurethral resection of prostate
U	Units
UA	Urinanalysis
UBO	Unidentified bright object
UGI	Upper gastrointestinal
UGIS	Upper GI series
URI	Upper respiratory illness
US	Ultrasound
USPTF	US preventive task force
UTI	Urinary tract infection
UV	Ultraviolet
UVA	Ultraviolet A
UVB	Ultraviolet B
UUB	Urine urobilinogen
vag	vaginally
val	Valine
VCUG	Vesico-urethrogram
VDRL	Serologic test for syphilis ("Venereal Disease Research Lab")
VF	Ventricular fibrillation
Vfib	Ventricular fibrillation
VIP	Vasoactive intestinal peptide
vit	Vitamin
VLDL	Very low density lipoprotein
VMA	Vanillymandelic acid
vol	Volume
V/Q	Ventilation/perfusion
VSD	Ventricular septal defect
VT	Ventricular tachycardia
Vtach	Ventricular tachycardia
V-ZIG	Varicella-zoster immune globulin
W/s	Watt/seconds
w/u	Work up
wbc	White blood cells or white blood count
wgt	Weight

wk	Week(s)
WNL	Within normal limits
WPW	Wolff-Parkinson-White Syndrome (short PR interval)
xmatch	Crossmatch
yr	Year(s)
ZE	Zollinger-Ellison syndrome
Zn	Zinc
>	More than
>>	Much more than
<	Less than
<<	Much less than
→	Leads to (eg, in a chemical reaction)

Journal Abbreviations

ACP J Club	American College of Physicians Journal Club
Am Fam Phys	American Family Physician
Am J Clin Path	American Journal of Clinical Pathology
Am J Dis Child	American J of Diseases of Childhood
Am J Med	American Journal of Medicine
Am J Obgyn	American Journal of Obstetrics and Gynecology
Am J Pub Hlth	American Journal of Public Health
Am J Respir Crit Care Med	American Journal of Respiratory and Critical Care Medicine
Am J Resp Med	American Journal of Respiratory Medicine
Am J Trop Med Hyg	American Journal of Tropical Medicine and Hygiene
Am Rev Resp Dis	American Review of Respiratory Disease
Ann EM	Annals of Emergency Medicine
Ann IM	Annals of Internal Medicine
Ann Neurol	Annals of Neurology
Annu Rev Public Health	Annual Review of Public Health
Arch Derm	Archives of Dermatology
Arch Pediatr Adolesc Med	Archives of Pediatric and Adolescent Medical Diseases
Aviat Space Env Med	Aviation Space and Environmental Medicine
BMJ	British Medical Journal
Bull Rheum Dis	Bulletin of Rheumatic Diseases
Can Med Assoc J	Canadian Medical Association Journal

Chemother	Chemotherapeutics
CID	Clinical Infectious Disease
Circ	Circulation
Crit Care Med	Critical Care Medicine
Curr Clin Top Inf Dis	Current Clinical Topics in Infectious Diseases
Diab Care	Diabetes Care
Emerging Inf Dis	Emerging Infectious Diseases
Epidem Rev	Epidemiology Review
FDA Bul	Federal Drug Administration Bulletin
GE	Gastroenterology
Inf Contr Hosp Epidem	Infection Control and Hospital Epidemiology
Inf Dis Clin NA	Infectious Disease Clinics of North America
Jama	Journal of the American Medical Association
J Am Acad Derm	Journal of the American Academy of Dermatology
J Clin Epidem	Journal of Clinical Epidemiology
J Clin Micro	Journal of Clinical Microbiology
J Fam Pract	Journal of Family Practice
J Gen Intern Med	Journal of General Internal Medicine
J Infect	Journal of Infection
J Infect Dis	Journal of Infectious Disease
J Intern Med	Journal of Internal Medicine
J Lab Clin Med	Journal of Laboratory and Clinical Medicine
J Peds	Journal of Pediatrics
J Travel Med	Journal of Travel Medicine
Mayo Clin Proc	Mayo Clinic Proceedings
Med	Medicine
Med Clin NA	Medical Clinics of North America

Med J Austral	Medical Journal of Australia
Med Let	Medical Letter
Mil Med	Military Medicine
Mmwr	CDC Morbidity and Mortality Weekly Review
Nat Hist	Natural History
Nejm	New England Journal of Medicine
Neurol	Neurology
Ophthalm	Ophthalmology
Ped Infect Dis J	Pediatric Infectious Disease Journal
Ped Rev	Pediatric Review
Peds	Pediatrics
Post Grad Med J	Postgraduate Medicine Journal
Q J Med	Quarterly Journal of Medicine
Rev Inf Dis	Review of Infectious Disease
Rx Let	Prescribers Letter
S African Med J	South African Medical Journal
Trans Roy Soc Trop Med Hyg	Transactions of the Royal Society of Tropical Medicine and Hygiene
Trav Med Adv	Travel Medicine Adviser
Trop Geog Med	Tropical and Geographic Medicine
Trop Med Int Health	Tropical Medicine and International Health
West J Med	Western Journal of Medicine
Wild Env Med	Wilderness and Environmental Medicine

Section I

EPIDEMIOLOGY OF
TRAVEL MEDICINE

1 Overview of Risk

Death rates among travelers not higher than nontravelers, but travelers likely to be a healthier subset of national populations (J Travel Med 2000;7:227); of all deaths in Canadians traveling abroad, 60% termed "natural" (w cardiovascular the most common dx)
- 25% due to accidents (mostly vehicular), 13% due to homicide/suicide (J Travel Med 2000;7:227); median age 43 yr (av 56 yr)
- Among Peace Corps volunteers (1962–1983), unintentional injuries caused 70% of deaths (mostly mvas, esp motorcycles; riding in open trucks also implicated); suicide/homicide 9%; infectious diseases only 4% (Jama 1985;254:1326)
- U.S. travelers (seen at a travel clinic before trip) to developing countries experienced the following: diarrhea (40%), respiratory illness (26%), skin disorders (8%), acute mountain sickness (6%), motion sickness (5%), accidents and injuries (5%), isolated febrile episodes (3%); 26% remained ill on return (J Travel Med 2000;7:259)
- Similar data reported for European travelers to tropics w 10% seeking medical consultation abroad (J Travel Med 1997;4:61)
- Overall w international travel: emergency medical evacuation 0.01–0.1%; fatalities in 0.001%/month (JID 1987;156:84)

RISK FOR TRAVELERS

Duration of trip and destination (see Fig. 1.1) are important (J Travel Med 2000;7:259); rates of illness/injury higher w young age (ie, college, etc.), adventurous travel (Swiss data show fatality rate of 0.015% in trekkers to Nepal vs 0.0003% in travelers to U.S.; Dupont et al, 1999).

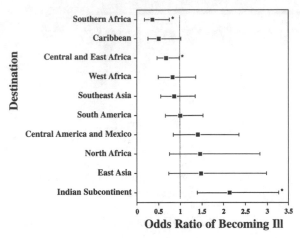

Figure 1.1. Odds ratio of developing illness by destination using a logistic regression analysis, with 95% confidence levels indicated. (Reproduced with permission from J Travel Med 2000;7:259.)

* p <.05.

INFECTIOUS DISEASE RISK

Traveler's diarrhea in 1/3–1/2 tropical travelers; malaria depends on destination and use of chemoprophylaxis; overall 0.4%, but in W. Africa 2.4%/mo (Lancet 1993;341:1299); hepatitis A 0.3%/mo to 1.5%/mo in backpackers (Jama 1994;272:885); typhoid 0.003%/mo (JID 1987;156:84); cholera 0.0003%/mo. See Fig. 1.2. (J Travel Med 1995;2:154)

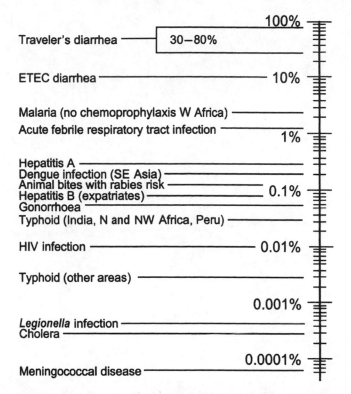

Figure 1.2. Monthly incidence rates of health problems during stay in developing countries. ETEC, enterotoxigenic *Escherichia coli*. (Reproduced with permission from CID 2000;30:809.)

ACCIDENT/INJURY RISK

Motor vehicle injuries/deaths occur at greater frequency w foreign travel than at home (Ann Emergency Med 1991;20:6), and account for 26% of mortality in U.S. travelers abroad. In Peace Corps volunteers, 1/3 of motor vehicle accidents related to motorcycle use (Jama 1985;254:1326). Drownings are second most common cause of accident related death among U.S. citizen travelers. Suicide is an important cause of death in Peace Corps (13% of deaths in Jama study), but accounted for only 3% of deaths among U.S. citizen travelers as a group.

Section II

PREVENTION OF TRAVEL-RELATED ILLNESS

2 Components of Pretravel Visit

KEY FACTORS

- Assessment of itinerary (where and when)
- Assessment of purpose of trip (what)
- Assessment of medical hx
- Required/recommended vaccinations (see Chapter 3)
- Malaria prevention/chemoprophylaxis (see Chapter 4)
- Traveler's diarrhea management plan (see Chapters 5, 16.47)
- Environmental considerations (ie, altitude, etc.) (see Chapter 7)
- Medical illness contingencies (insurance, etc.)

Assessment of itinerary:
- Include assessment of countries to be visited (see Appendix 1)
- Urban vs rural travel
- Expected duration of trip and departure date
- Border crossings

Assessment of purpose:
- Business vs recreational
- Visits to relatives or friends
- Unusual activities planned (hiking, snorkeling, etc)

Medical hx:
- Active medical illness (ie, diabetes – see sect 9.4)
- Past medical hx (esp childhood diseases, jaundice, seizures, psychiatric illness)
- Immunosuppression (HIV, steroid use, etc.) (see section 9.2)
- Medications
- Allergies (medicines, bees/wasps, eggs)
- Pregnancy (current or anticipated), breast feeding (see section 9.1)

Required/recommended vaccinations (see Chapter 3):
- Required for entry to some countries: yellow fever
- Often recommended: update Td, other routine immuniz if needed (MMR, varicella)
- Hepatitis A, hepatitis B, typhoid, polio depending on risk assessment/immuniz hx
- Less frequently recommended: meningococcal, pre-exposure rabies, Japanese encephalitis, cholera, Lyme
- Unavailable in U.S.: plague, anthrax, tick-borne encephalitis vaccines
- Consider risk/benefit, contraindications, timing (see Chapter 3)

Malaria prevention:
- Assess risk based on itinerary/activities (see Chapter 4)
- For those at risk, educate re: preventive measures
- Consider options for chemoprophylaxis (see Chapter 4)
- Counsel on importance of evaluation of all fevers on return

Traveler's diarrhea:
- Provide information on food/water safety (see Chapter 5)
- Provide information on management of traveler's diarrhea
- Give antibiotic for self rx w information if appropriate (see Chapters 5, 16.47)

Environmental considerations:
- Prevention/rx altitude illness (see Chapter 7)
- Provide information on prevention of arthropod bites, etc.

For prolonged/remote trips:
- Review traveler's medical kit
- Discuss health hazards particular to setting
- Discuss heath contingency plans

Contingencies:
- Provide information on travel insurance/health care abroad

3 Immunizations

3.1 OVERVIEW

Med Let 1999;41:39; Med Clini N Am 1999;83:903
Vaccines are generally divided into three categories: routine immunizations (the usual childhood vaccines), which should be up-to-date regardless of travel; required immunizations, which are those vaccines required for entry into certain countries by the World Health Organization (WHO); and recommended immunizations, which are vaccines that should be offered to travelers to decrease the risk of contracting certain infectious diseases. Recommended vaccines can be of great benefit to travelers and usually require a pretrip consultation and sufficient time prior to departure to ensure adequate protection. Legal requirements (required vaccines) for entry and epidemiologic conditions in different countries vary from time-to-time and may be unpredictable. Up-to-date resources should be used routinely (CDC Blue Sheet at <hhtp//www.cdc.gov/travel/index.htm> or by fax at 1-888-CDC-FAXX). Presently, the vaccine against yellow fever is the only WHO-required vaccine (see Figs. 3.1A and 3.1B)

Most vaccines for travel fall into the recommended category and decisions regarding their use will need to be individualized depending on destination, style and duration of travel, and underlying host factors. Often, health plans do not provide adequate coverage for vaccines, making them discretionary expenditures for the traveler. Nonetheless, these vaccines prevent diseases such as hepatitis A, rabies, meningococcal meningitis, and others that are prevalent in developing nations and pose serious threats to the traveler. Therefore, recommended vaccines should be considered a high priority for many travelers. It is important to emphasize that developing nations (the destination of many travelers) have not developed routine hygiene standards and water purification, resulting in incr risk hepatitis A, typhoid, other enterically transmitted infections. In addition, sewage removal can not be assured and arthropod-borne diseases, such as malaria, dengue, and yellow fever, are prevalent. Simply stated, the transmission of many infectious diseases rarely seen in the U.S. occurs in developing nations. Vaccines offer an effective strategy to avoid the morbidity and possible mortality associated with some of these infections.

3.2 GENERAL PRINCIPLES

Timing of vaccines: Some vaccines require more than one dose for protection; the use of multiple reduced doses given at less than minimum intervals may not be effective; except for oral typhoid vaccine, it is unnecessary to restart an interrupted series of a vaccine or toxoid or to add extra doses; some vaccines require boosters to maintain protection

Simultaneous administration: All commonly used vaccines can be administered on the same day on separate sites if possible; yellow fever and cholera vaccines should be separated by 3 weeks, if possible; live viral vaccines should ideally be given on the same day or separated by 28 days to maximize immune responses; avoid giving immune globulin preparations and some live virus vaccines (ie, MMR, varicella) at the same time; see Table 3.6 for specific recommended intervals

Acute illness: Persons with severe illness should be vaccinated as soon as their condition improves; this precaution is to avoid superimposing adverse effects; mild illness should not delay needed vaccines; the immune response will still be effective; antibiotics interfere with live oral bacterial vaccines, such as oral typhoid, and should not be given simultaneously

Recording vaccines: Record date, dose, site, lot number, and vaccine type; provide the traveler with a written record of vaccine administration in an international certificate of immunizations booklet (see Fig. 3.2); yellow fever vaccine requires an official seal at legally authorized sites

Adverse events: Report all possible adverse events to "Vaccine Adverse Events Reporting System" (VAERS) 1-800-822-7967; immune-compromised or pregnant patients generally should not receive live virus vaccines.

3.3 SUMMARY OF VACCINES

A. ROUTINE VACCINES

Polio:
- After completion of primary series CDC recommends an additional dose in adult life if traveling to a polio-endemic country

Tetanus/diphtheria: After completion of a primary series, once every 10 years.

Measles: CDC recommends a dose of measles vaccine for nonimmune persons born in or after 1957 who have not had two doses on or after the first birthday

Hepatitis B: Consider for long-term travelers (staying >6 months) going to intermediate or high-prevalence areas and ANY short-term travelers who may have incr risk for contact with blood or body fluids

Influenza: Influenza endemic in tropics, exposure on planes—consider for high-risk areas

Pneumococcal: Consider for all usual indications as in U.S.; recognize exposure may be increased w travel due to crowding during transportation, etc.

Varicella: Consider for nonimmune persons

IMMUNIZATIONS

B. TRAVEL VACCINES

Cholera (whole cell vaccine): Rarely recommended (low vaccine efficacy); clinical dx of cholera is rare in travelers; new vaccine may improve efficacy (see 3.8)

Hepatitis A: Consider for all travelers except those traveling to developed countries in Europe, Japan, Australia, New Zealand, or Canada

Japanese encephalitis: Should generally be considered for travelers who will be visiting 30 days or longer to rural areas in all of Asia, the Indian Subcontinent, and Western Pacific where JEV is present and during the season of transmission; however, due to allergic rxns and rarity of clinical JE in travelers, risk/benefit of this vaccine more complex than for most other recommended travel vaccines; see 20.2 (JEV)

Meningococcal meningitis:
- Consider if traveling during December–June to the subSaharan Meningitis Belt (see 16.27)
- May be required for travelers to Saudi Arabia during the Hajj, or to other areas during outbreaks

Plague: Rarely recommended and no longer routinely available

Rabies (preexposure): Consider for travelers who might be exposed to wild or domestic animals through work or recreation, especially for travel to remote areas where postexposure rx not readily available, or for long-term travelers to developing countries

Tickborne encephalitis:
- Not available in the U.S.
- Use insect repellent to minimize risk

Typhoid fever: Consider for travelers staying in areas of questionable sanitation, adventurous travelers, long-term travelers (>3–4 wks) and all travelers to the Indian subcontinent

Yellow fever: Recommended for travel to endemic areas—may be required for entry to many countries of Africa, So America

Lyme disease: Rarely used for travel—outdoor exposure in risk areas in northeast, midwestern U.S.

Smallpox: No longer available; smallpox eradicated

Typhus: Vaccine discontinued

Required Vaccines

3.4 YELLOW FEVER VACCINE

Mmwr 1990;39:1; Jama 1996;276:1157

Disease: Mosquito borne viral disease, flu-like illness to severe hepatitis, and hemorrhagic fever (see 20.16)

Indications: Travelers to rural tropical So America and SubSaharan Africa where YF is endemic (see Fig. 3.1); required for entry to some countries, including some Asian/Pacific (nonendemic) countries when hx of departure from endemic area

Vaccine: Live attenuated virus (17D strain) prepared in eggs; 0.5 mL SC—effective 10 d after inoculation; contraindicated in egg allergy, children <9 months, pregnant and lactating women, immune compromised; if contraindicated, but required for entry, send a letter on physician letterhead stating reasons for contraindications; only available at approved yellow fever vaccination centers (see designated list available through state/local health departments); certificate (see Fig. 3.2) valid 10 d after vaccination; avoid giving w/in 3 wks of cholera vaccine

Immunogenicity/efficacy: 98% for >10 yrs; only 1 known case has occurred in a vaccinated traveler

Boosters: Recommended q 10 yrs (though immunity from single injection may persist for >30 yrs)

Side Effects: Generally mild, 2–5% low grade temp, 5–10 d after vaccine; reaction is debilitating in <0.2%; immediate hypersensitivity in <1/million doses; usually in someone w egg allergy; several cases of vaccine-related encephalitis have occurred when given to infants (usually <4 mo); avoid giving within 3 weeks of cholera vaccine, if possible

Contraindications: Hx egg allergy; children <9 mos, pregnancy, immune compromised; note that no actual cases of encephalitis, etc. reported in immune compromised, but theoretical risk exists; CDC states that vaccine appears safe if only low-dose steroids (ie, 10 mg/d) or short course (<2 wks); asymptomatic HIV pts may be vaccinated (see 9.2); response may be diminished; for more information, call CDC at (970)-221-6400.

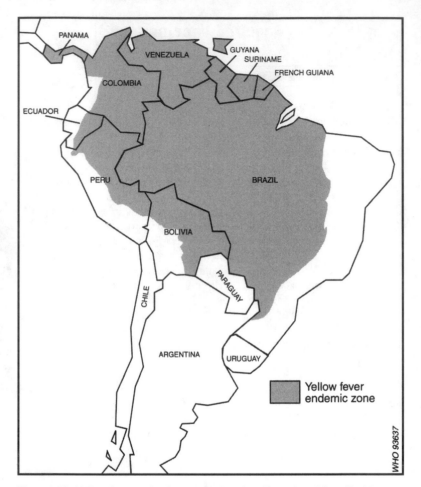

Figure 3.1A. Yellow fever endemic zones in America. (Reproduced from Health Information for International Travel, CDC.)

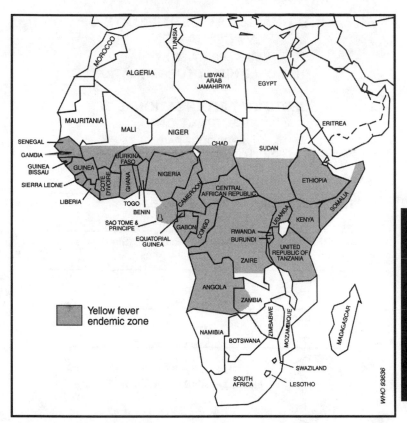

Figure 3.1B. Yellow fever endemic zones in Africa. (Reproduced from Health Information for International Travel, CDC.)

According to WHO, vaccine has been used in pregnancy at >6 mo if risk is of exposure is unavoidable, but not approved for this use by FDA

Vaccine handling: Must be stored between 5°C and 30°C; preferably frozen until reconstitution; once reconstituted, unused vaccine must be discarded after 1–2 hr

INTERNATIONAL CERTIFICATE OF VACCINATION

AS APPROVED BY
THE WORLD HEALTH ORGANIZATION

CERTIFICAT INTERNATIONAL DE VACCINATION

APPROUVÉ PAR
L'ORGANISATION MONDIALE DE LA SANTÉ

TRAVELER'S NAME–NOM DU VOYAGEUR

ADDRESS–ADRESSE (Number–Numéro)   (Street–Rue)

(City–Ville)

(County–Département)   (State–État)

**U.S. DEPARTMENT OF
HEALTH AND HUMAN SERVICES**

PUBLIC HEALTH SERVICE

PHS–731 (REV.11-91)

THIS CERTIFICATE IS VALID only if the vaccine used has been approved by the World Health Organization and if the vaccinating center has been designated by the health administration for the country in which the center is situated.

THE VALIDITY OF THIS CERTIFICATE shall extend for a period of 10 years, beginning 10 days after the date of vaccination or, in the event of a revaccination, within such period of 10 years from the date of that revaccination.

This certificate must be hand signed by a medical practitioner or other person authorized by the national health administration. An official signature stamp is not acceptable.

Any amendment of this certificate, or erasure, or failure to complete any part of it, may render it invalid.

Figure 3.2. International certificate of vaccination.

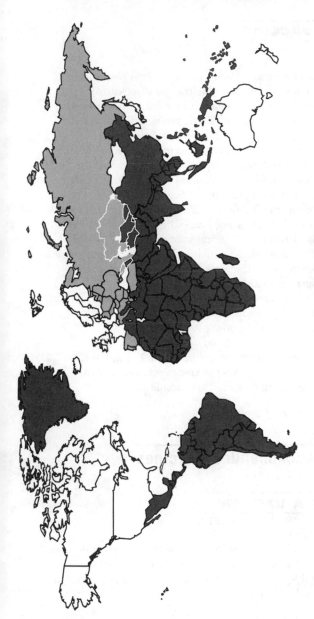

Anti-HAV Prevalence

■ High

▨ Intermediate

□ Low

Figure 3.3. Geographic distribution of Hepatitis A infection. (Reproduced from Health Information for International Travel, CDC.)

IMMUNIZATIONS

3.5 CHOLERA VACCINE

CID 2000;31:561

Disease: Acute intestinal infection from toxin of *Vibrio cholerae* (see 16.13); very low risk for routine travelers (incidence <0.000003/mo); H_2 blockers, antacids incr risk of infection

Indications: Generally not recommended; the whole cell inactivated vaccine (cholera vaccine USP) is not very effective and is reactogenic; requirement for cholera vaccine dropped by WHO—occasional countries still might require—considered in those on H_2 blockers, antacids visiting high-risk areas or in persons living in highly endemic areas w/o access to medical care

Vaccine: Killed whole cell vaccine only vaccine available in U.S. (see Table 3.1); new oral vaccines not licensed in U.S., but available in Europe, Canada; attenuated live oral vaccine (CVD 103-HgR) appears more efficacious; inactivated oral (whole cell-beta subunit) has 50–60% protective efficacy over 3 yrs, and offers some protection against toxigenic *E. coli* (see Table 3.1)

Efficacy: 50% in reducing illness from 01-type disease; does not protect against cholera 0139 (Bengal) strain (no current vaccine is protective against Bengal strain)

Booster: Doses recommended every 6 mo

Side effects: Pain, erythema induration common for 1–2 d; fever, malaise, ha on occasion; serious adverse events are very rare

Contraindications: Prior allergic rxn to this vaccine

Recommended Vaccines

3.6 HEPATITIS A VACCINE

Mmwr 1999;48(RR 12):1

Disease: Enterically transmitted viral disease—mild to severe; fulminant disease w 27 deaths/1000 cases over age 50; most common vaccine preventable travel related illness; risk 0.3–2% per mo in unprotected travelers (see 20.7)

Indications: All travelers to the developing world (see Fig. 3.3) and others w preexisting liver disease, HIV, etc. Consider prevaccination serologic screening for immunity in persons born prior to 1945, or w hx unexplained jaundice, or residence >1 yr in developing countries (J Trav Med 1999;6:107; Jama 1994;275:885)

Vaccine: Two licensed formalin-inactivated viral particle vaccines offering high level of protection; a combined hep A/B formulation has recently been approved in U.S.; dosing as in Tables 3.2 and 3.3

Immunogenicity/efficacy: Antibodies develop in 32%–80% at 2 wks, 95% at one mo; nearly 100% children protected after 1 dose (Jama 1994;271:328)

Booster: 2 doses (usually given 6 or more mo apart) provides long-term protection; for combined hep A/B vaccine, 3 doses (0, 1, 6 mo); 2 hep A vaccines (ie, Vaqta, Havrix) appear interchangeable for booster response (Vaccine 2001;19:1416); optimal timing for booster is 12–60 mo (Vaccine 2001;19:399)

Side effects: Mild—soreness at site, ha 20%–45% (CID 2001;32:396); anaphylaxis rare; overall well tolerated—safety in pregnancy is unknown, but it is generally recommended if risk of disease is significant; rare multisystemic post-vaccination syndrome reported in elderly travelers (Lancet 2000;358:98)

Contraindications: Allergy to vaccine or aluminum

Prevaccination: Serologic testing cost-effective in pts born before 1945 or w hx jaundice

Vaccine handling: Should not be frozen

Prevent: Immune globulin is protective if vaccine is not given (see Table 3.4) or combined w vaccine if trip w/in 4 wks; however, often not available; efficacy of immune globulin is 85%. Vaccine is preferred—hepatitis A virus is inactivated by boiling or cooking; avoid contaminated food and water

Table 3.1. Cholera vaccine

Doses (mL)	Intradermal route*	Subcutaneous or intramuscular route			Comments
	≥5 yr of age	6 mo–4 yr of age	5–10 yr of age	>10 yr of age	
Primary series: 1 and 2	0.2	0.2	0.3	0.5	Give 1 wk to >1 mo apart
Booster	0.2	0.2	0.3	0.5	1 dose every 6 mo

* Higher levels of protection (antibody) may be achieved in children <5 yr of age if vaccine is administered by the subcutaneous or intramuscular routes.
Adapted from Health Information for International Travel, Centers for Disease Control.

Table 3.2. Recommended doses of Havrix*

Group	Age (yr)	Dose (EL.U.)[†]	Volume (mL)	Number of doses	Schedule (mo)[§]
Children and adolescents[¶]	2–18	720	0.5	2	0.6–12
Adults	>18	1440	1.0	2	0.6–12

* Hepatitis A vaccine, inactivated, SmithKline Beecham.
[†] EL.U = ELISA units.
[§] 0 months represents timing of the initial dose; subsequent numbers represent months after the initial dose.
[¶] An alternate formulation and schedule (3 doses) are available for children and adolescents, consisting of 360 EL.U per 0.5 mL dose at 0, 1, and 6–12 mo of age.
Adapted from Health Information for International Travel, Centers for Disease Control.

Table 3.3. Recommended doses of Vaqta*

Group	Age (yr)	Dose (EL.U.)[†]	Volume (mL)	Number of doses	Schedule (mo)[§]
Children and adolescents	2–7	25 U	0.5	2	0.6–18
Adults	>17	50 U	1.0	2	0.6–12

* Hepatitis A vaccine, inactivated, Merck & Company, Inc.
[†] Units.
[§] 0 months represents timing of the initial dose; subsequent numbers represent months after the initial dose.
Adapted from Health Information for International Travel, Centers for Disease Control.

Table 3.4. Immune globulin for protection against viral hepatitis A

Length of stay	Body weight		Dose volume (mL)*	Comments
	lb	kg[†]		
Short-term travel (<3 mo)	<50	<23	0.5	Dose volume depends on body weight and length of stay
	50–100	23–45	1.0	
	>100	>45	2.0	
Long-term travel (3–5 mo)	<22	<10	0.5	
	<50	<23	1.0	
	50–100	23–45	2.5	
	>100	>45	5.0	

* For intramuscular injection.
[†] kg = approximately 2.2 lb.
Adapted from Health Information for International Travel, Centers for Disease Control.

IMMUNIZATIONS

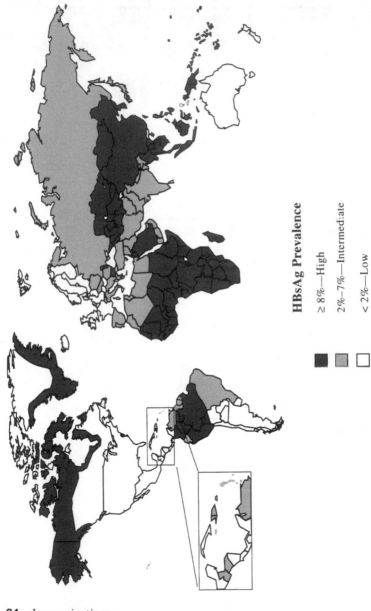

HBsAg Prevalence

■ ≥ 8%—High

▨ 2%–7%—Intermediate

□ < 2%—Low

Figure 3.4. Geographic distribution of Hepatitis B prevalence. (Reproduced from Health Information for International Travel, CDC.)

3.7 HEPATITIS B VACCINE

Nejm 1997;336:196

Disease: Viral infection of the liver—asymptomatic to fulminant—chronic infection (5–10%); blood borne and sexual transmission (see 20.8)

Indications: High-risk travelers including health care workers, long-term travelers to highly endemic areas, and anyone who might have sexual contact with new partner (see Fig. 3.4); risk of hep B in travelers ranges from 0.05–0.01/mo (J Travel Med 2001;8:53)

Vaccine: Recombinant vaccine derived from envelope protein (Engerix and Recombivax)—3 dose series—im 0, 1, 6–12 months—routine childhood vaccine, avoid gluteal injection; accelerated schedules 0, 1, 2 months with f/u at 12 mo an option for travelers (JID 1989;160:766); shorter regimens (0, 4, 28 d; 0, 7, 21 d) may also be effective (75%) if necessary (J Travel Med 1995;2:213); boost at 12 mo; similar effectiveness reported w combined hep A/B vaccine; these two vaccines are interchangeable; see Table 3.5

Immunogenicity/efficacy: Protective serum titers in 90–95% after 3 doses in healthy recipients; 70–80% after 2 doses; larger doses may be chosen for immune-suppressed individuals

Booster: None except in setting of exposure and inadequate antibody level (<10 IU); even individuals who lose antibody are thought to be protected

Table 3.5. Recommended doses of currently licensed hepatitis B vaccines

Group	Dose (µg)	
	Recombivax HB*	Engerix-B*
All infants (regardless of mother's HBsAg status) and children birth to 19 yr of age	5	10
Adults ≥20 yr	10	20
Dialysis patients and other immunocompromised persons	40[†]	40[§]

* Both vaccines are routinely administered in a 3-dose series. Engerix-B also has been licensed for a 4-dose series administered at 0, 1, 2, and 12 mo.

[†] Special formulation (40 µg in 1.0 mL).

[§] Two 1.0-mL doses given at one site, in a 4-dose schedule at 0, 1, 2, 6 mo.

Adapted from Health Information for International Travel, Centers for Disease Control.

Side effects: Well tolerated—sore arm—20%, mild systemic symptoms 5%; rare reports of anaphylaxis (Jama 1994;271:1602)
Contraindications: Hypersensitivity to yeast, other vaccine components
Handling: Do not freeze
Precautions: Avoid contact with body fluids and secretions—safe sexual practices or abstinence

3.8 MEASLES VACCINE

Mmwr 1998;47:8; Jama 1997;277:1952
Disease: Rubeola—acute viral illness with rash, multiple possible complications; prevalent in the developing world, where it accounts for 10% global mortality
Indication: Risk outside U.S. may be high; varies from 0.1 to 8/million travelers; common disease all over the world, but marked decline in imported cases from Latin America. Indicated for all without proof of vaccine or disease; note that a single MMR vaccination may not be protective for adults
Vaccine: Live attenuated vaccine—either MMR (measles, mumps, rubella) or single monovalent antigen; anyone born after 1956 needs 2 doses unless prior hx measles, positive measles serology (EIA, ELISA)—routine childhood vaccine (MMR); children 6–11 mo should receive the vaccine then be revaccinated at 15 mo; see Table 3.6 for suggested timing of intervals between use of immune globulin preparations and live measles vaccine
Efficacy: 95% at greater than 12 mo age
Booster: None after 2 doses
Side effects: Fever and rash 5%, 7–12 days after vaccine; self-limited; rare anaphylaxis (<1 case/million); transient lymphadenopathy, parotitis w rubella component; this may cause arthritis (self-limited) in 10% (Am J Epidemiol 1982;118:19); rare encephalopathy (1 case per 2 million)
Contraindications: Do not use in immunocompromised—avoid in pregnancy—postpone if possible with moderate to acute illness —administer at least 14 days before immune globulins
In HIV positive pts, rare giant cell pneumonia due to MMR use (Ann IM 1998;129:104); diminished antibody responses if low CD4; can give MMR if necessary to pts w/o sx and CD4 >200

Table 3.6. Suggested intervals between administration of immune globulin preparations for various indications and vaccines containing live measles virus*

Indication	Dose (including mg of IgG/kg)	Suggested interval before measles vaccination
RSV monoclonal antibody (Synagis)[†]	15 mg/kg im	None
Tetanus (TIG)	250 units (10 mg IgG/kg) im	3 months
Hepatitis A (IG)		
Contact prophylaxis	0.02 mL/kg (3.3 mg IgG/kg) im	3 months
International travel	0.06 mL/kg (10 mg IgG/kg) im	3 months
Hepatitis B prophylaxis (HBIG)	0.06 mL/kg (10 mg IgG/kg) im	3 months
Rabies prophylaxis (HRIG)	20 IU/kg (22 mg IgG/kg) im	4 months
Varicella prophylaxis (VZIG)	125 units/10kg (20–40 mg IgG/kg) im (maximum 625 units)	5 months
Measles prophylaxis (IG)		
Normal contact	0.25 mL/kg (40 mg IgG/kg) im	5 months
Immunocompromised contact[§]	0.50 mL/kg (80 mg IgG/kg) im	6 months
Blood transfusion		
Red blood cells (RBCs), washed	10 mL/kg (negligible IgG/kg) iv	None
RBCs, adenine-saline added	10 mL/kg (10 mg/IgG/kg) iv	3 months
Packed RBCs (Hct 65%)[¶]	10 mL/kg (60 mg/IgG/kg) iv	6 months
Whole blood (Hct 35–50%)[¶]	10 mL/kg (80–100 mg/IgG/kg) iv	6 months
Plasma/platelet products	10 mL/kg (160 mg/IgG/kg) iv	7 months

Table 3.6. *(cont'd)*

Indication	Dose (including mg of IgG/kg)	Suggested interval before measles vaccination
Cytomegalovirus prophylaxis (CMV IGIV)	150 mg/kg (maximum)	6 months
Respiratory syncytial virus prophylaxis (RSV IGIV)	750 mg/kg	9 months
Intravenous Immune Globulin (IGIV)		
IGIV, Replacement therapy	300–400 mg/kg iv¶	8 months
IGIV, ITP**	400 mg/kg iv	8 months
IGIV, ITP**	1000 mg/kg iv	10 months
IGIV, Kawasaki disease	2 g/kg iv	11 months

* This table is not intended to be used for determining the correct indications and dosage for the use of IG preparations. Unvaccinated persons may not be fully protected against measles during the entire suggested interval, and additional doses of IG and/or measles vaccine may be indicated following measles exposure. The concentration of measles antibody in a particular IG preparation can vary by lot. The rate of antibody clearance following receipt of an IG preparation can also vary. The recommended intervals are extrapolated from an estimated half-life of 30 days for passively acquired antibody and an observed interference with the immune response to measles vaccine for 5 months following a dose of 80 IgG/kg.

† Contains only antibody to respiratory syncytial virus (RSV).

§ Measles vaccination is recommended for children with HIV infection but is contraindicated in patients with congenital disorders of the immune system.

¶ Assumes a serum IgG concentration of 16 mg/mL.

** Immune (formerly, idiopathic) thrombocytopenic purpura.

Adapted from Health Information for International Travel, Centers for Disease Control.

Prevent: If nonimmune, hard to prevent—if exposed, gamma globulin vaccination preferred strategy

3.9 MENINGOCOCCAL VACCINE

Mmwr 1997;46:1; Nejm 2001;344:1378

Disease: Acute bacterial infection with meningitis, high morbidity and mortality, rare in travelers (see 16.27)

Indication: Travel to Sahel (SubSaharan Africa) or areas with known epidemics where attack rates may reach 1%; check w CDC (404-332-4559); see Fig. 3.5 (Meningitis Belt); also consider in pts w splenectomy

Vaccine: Quadrivalent single dose vaccine sero group A, C, Y, W-I35 (menomune); purified capsular polysaccharide; no vaccine for serotype B; antibiotic prophylaxis for unimmunized close contacts of infectious cases; no benefit at age <2; (new conjugated meningococcal vaccines may be more effective; not yet available); single-dose vials now available

Immunogenicity/efficacy: Protective efficacy of 70–100% for groups A, C; unknown for Y, W135, though both are immunogenic

Booster: Every 3–5 yrs for adults; revaccinate 2–3 yrs for childen <4

Side effects: Infrequent and mild, localized pain, 1–2% mild fever

Contraindications: Allergic reactions to prior doses (contains thiomersal); category C in pregnancy

Prevent: People-to-people exposure makes precaution difficult; antibiotic prophylaxis (ciprofloxacin 500 mg once, rifampin 300 mg bid × 2 d, or ceftriaxone 125 mg once)

3.10 JAPANESE B ENCEPHALITIS VACCINE

Lancet 1996;348:341

Disease: Mosquito-borne flavivirus (see 20.2) endemic in rural Asia, especially near pig farming areas w associated rice paddies; most infections asymptomatic (inapparent : apparent disease = 300 : 1) but serious encephalitis/deaths in up to 40% of symptomatic cases; seasonal transmission (see Table 3.7)

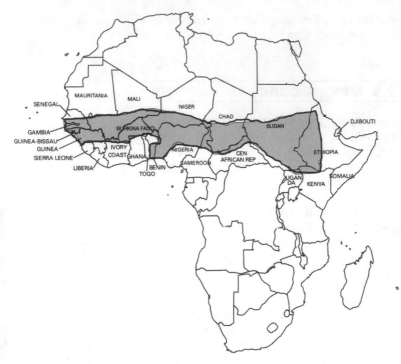

Figure 3.5. Sub-Saharan meningitis belt. (Reproduced from Morbidity and Mortality Weekly Report, CDC, 1997.)

Indications: Travelers to rural Asia with extensive (>1 month) unprotected outdoor activity, especially in summer and autumn in endemic areas with extensive mosquito content; disease in travelers is rare (<2 cases/yr in U.S. travelers/military personnel), and allergic side effects of vaccine make judicious use of vaccine appropriate, especially in persons w multiple allergies

Vaccine: Formalin inactivated mouse brain derived vaccine (Table 3.8) JE-VAX—dose adults 1 mL, 3 shot series, 2 doses 1 wk apart gives reasonable short-term protection; a live attenuated vaccine is in use in China

Immunogenicity/efficacy: 100% seroconversion by third dose; 80% at second dose

Table 3.7. Risk of Japanese encephalitis, by country, region, and season

Country	Affected areas/jurisdictions	Transmission season	Comments
Australia	Islands of Torres Strait	Probably year-round transmission risk	Localized outbreak in Torres Strait in 1995 and sporadic cases in 1998 in Torres Strait and on mainland Australia at Cape York Peninsula
Bangladesh	Few data, but probably widespread	Possibly July–December, as in northern India	Outbreak reported from Tangail district, Dacca division; sporadic cases in Rajshahi division
Bhutan	No data	No data	Not applicable
Brunei	Presumed to be sporadic–endemic as in Malaysia	Presumed year-round transmission	—
Cambodia	Presumed to be endemic–hyperendemic countrywide	Presumed to be May–October	Cases reported from refugee camps on Thai border
Hong Kong	Rare cases in new territories	April–October	Vaccine not routinely recommended
India	Reported cases from all states except Arunachal, Dadra, Daman, Diu, Gujarat, Himachal, Jammu, Kashmir, Lakshadweep, Meghalaya, Nagar Haveli, Orissa, Punjab, Rajasthan, Sikkim	*South India:* May–October in Goa; October–January in Tamil Nadu; August–December in Karnataka; second peak, April–June in Mandya district. *Andhra Pradesh:* September–December. *North India:* July–December	Outbreaks in West Bengal, Bihar, Karnataka, Tamil Nadu, Andhra Pradesh, Assam, Uttar Pradesh, Manipur, and Goa. Urban cases reported (eg, Lucknow)

Table 3.7. (cont'd)

Country	Affected areas/jurisdictions	Transmission season	Comments
Indonesia	Kalimantan, Bali, Nusa Tenggara, Sulawesi, Mollucas, and West Irian Jaya, Lombok	Probably year-round risk; varies by island; peak risks associated with rainfall, rice cultivation, and presence of pigs Peak periods of risk: November–March; June–July in some years	Human cases recognized on Bali and Java and possibly in Lombok
Japan*	Rare–sporadic cases on all islands except Hokkaido	June–September except Ryuku Islands (Okinawa) April–October	Vaccine not routinely recommended for travel to Tokyo and other major cities Enzootic transmission without human cases observed on Hokkaido
Korea	North Korea: no data South Korea: sporadic-endemic with occasional outbreaks	July–October	Last major outbreaks in 1982–1983; sporadic cases reported in 1994 and 1998
Laos	Presumed to be endemic–hyperendemic country-wide	Presumed to be May–October	No data available
Malaysia	Sporadic–endemic in all states of Peninsula, Sarawak, and probably Sabah	No seasonal pattern; year-round transmission	Most cases from Penang, Perak, Salangor, Johore, and Sarawak
Myanmar (Burma)	Presumed to be endemic–hyperendemic countrywide	Presumed to be May–October	Repeated outbreaks in Shan State in Chiang Mai Valley
Nepal	Hyperendemic in southern lowlands (Terai)	July–December	Vaccine not recommended for travelers visiting high-altitude areas only

Pakistan	May be transmitted in central deltas	Presumed to be June–January	Cases reported near Karachi; endemic areas overlap those for West Nile virus; lower Indus Valley may be an endemic transmission area

Country	Location	Transmission period	Notes
Pakistan	May be transmitted in central deltas	Presumed to be June–January	Cases reported near Karachi; endemic areas overlap those for West Nile virus; lower Indus Valley may be an endemic transmission area
Papua New Guinea	Normanby Islands and Western Province	Probably year-round risk	Localized sporadic cases
People's Republic of China	Cases in all provinces except Xizang (Tibet), Xinjiang, Qinghai. Hyperendemic in southern China; endemic–periodically epidemic in temperate areas	*Northern China:* May–September *Southern China:* April–October (Guangshi, Yunnan, Gwangdong, and Southern Fugian, Szechuan, Guizhou, Hunan, Jiangsi provinces)	Vaccine not routinely recommended for travelers to urban areas only
Philippines	Presumed to be endemic on all islands	Uncertain; speculations based on locations and agroecosystems: West Luzon, Mindoro, Negro Palowan: April–November Elsewhere: year-round, with greatest risk April–January	Outbreaks described in Nueva Ecija, Luzon, and Manila
Russia	Far eastern maritime areas south of Khabarousk	Peak period July–September	First human cases in 30 years recently reported
Singapore	Rare cases	Year-round transmission, with April peak	Vaccine not routinely recommended
Sri Lanka	Endemic in all but mountainous areas; periodically epidemic in northern and central provinces	October–January; secondary peak of enzootic transmission May–June	Recent outbreaks in central (Anuradhapura) and northwestern provinces
Taiwan*	Endemic, sporadic cases; island-wide	April–October, with a June peak	Cases reported in and around Taipei and the Kaohsiung-Pingtung river basins

IMMUNIZATIONS

Table 3.7. (*cont'd*)

Country	Affected areas/jurisdictions	Transmission season	Comments
Thailand	Hyperendemic in north; sporadic–endemic in south	May–October	Annual outbreaks in Chiang Mai Valley; sporadic cases in Bangkok suburbs
Vietnam	Endemic–hyperendemic in all provinces	May–October	Highest rates in and near Hanoi
Western Pacific	Two epidemics reported in Guam and Saipan since 1947	Uncertain; possibly September–January	Enzootic cycle may not be sustainable; epidemics may follow introductions of virus

* Local JE incidence rates may not accurately reflect risks to nonimmune visitors because of high immunization rates in local populations. Humans are incidental to the transmission cycle.

High levels of viral transmission may occur in the absence of human disease.

NOTE: Assessments are based on publications, surveillance reports, and personal correspondence. Extrapolations have been made from available data. Transmission patterns may change. Tsai TF, Yu Yx, Japanese encephalitis vaccines. In: Plotkin SA & Mortimer EA. *Vaccines.* 2nd ed., WB Saunders, Philadelphia 1994:671–713.

Adapted from Health Information for International Travel, Centers for Disease Control.

Table 3.8. Japanese encephalitis vaccine

Doses	Subcutaneous route (mL)		Comments
	1–2 years of age	≥3 years of age	^
Primary series 1, 2, and 3	0.5	1.0	Days 0, 7, 30
Booster*	1.0	1.0	1 dose at ≥36 months

* In vaccinees who have completed a 3-dose primary series, the full duration of protection is unknown; therefore, definitive recommendations cannot be given.
Adapted from Health Information for International Travel, Centers for Disease Control.

Booster: Every 3 yrs
Side effects:
- Allergic reactions including urticaria 0.5%, local systemic side effects 20%, anaphylaxis can occur
- Observe for 30 min after immunization; risk of rxn incr w allergy hx; in U.S. Marine Corps, rxn rate = 26/10,000 vaccinees; 2/3 were urticaria/angioedema; 1/3 were pruritus alone
- Median time to rxn is <48 hr dose 1, 96 hr dose 2 (CID 1997;24:265)

Contraindications: Allergic rxn to prior dose; not recommended in pregnancy

3.11 RABIES VACCINE (Pre-exposure)

Nejm 1993;329:1288
Disease: An acute fatal viral encephalomyelitis endemic worldwide, but w incr risk in South and Central America and parts of Asia, Africa (see 20.15); see also Table 3.9
Vaccine:
- Preexposure vaccination with human diploid cell rabies vaccine (HDCV), purified chick embryo cell vaccine (PCEC) or rabies vaccine adsorbed (RVA); see Table 3.10
- Preexposure immunization consists of 3 doses of HDCV, PCEC, or RVA, 1.0 mL, im (deltoid area), 1 each on days 0, 7, or 28; ONLY HDCV may be administered by the intradermal (id) dose/route (0.1 mL id on days 0, 7, and 21 or 28)

Table 3.9. Countries reporting no cases of rabies* 1996–1997

Region	Countries
Africa	Cape Verde; Libya[†]; Mauritius[†]; Reunion; Seychelles[†];
Americas	**North**: Bermuda; St. Pierre and Miquelon **Caribbean**: Most islands **South**: Uruguay
Asia	Bahrain; Brunei; Hong Kong; Japan; Kuwait; Malaysia (Malaysia-Sabah[†]); Maldives; Qatar; Singapore; Taiwan
Europe	Most, except Soviet Union
Oceania	Most of Pacific Oceania is "rabies-free"

* Bat rabies exists in some areas that are free of terrestrial rabies.
[†] Countries with classifications that may be considered provisional.
Adapted from Health Information for International Travel, Centers for Disease Control.

Table 3.10. Rabies immunization

I. PREEXPOSURE IMMUNIZATION. Preexposure immunization consists of three doses of HDCV, PCEC, or RVA, 1.0 mL, im (i.e., deltoid area), 1 each on days 0, 7, and 21 or 28. ONLY HDCV may be administered by the intradermal (id) dose/route (0.1 mL id on days 0, 7, and 21 or 28). If the traveler will be taking chloroquine or mefloquine for malaria chemoprophylaxis, the 3-dose series must be completed before antimalarials are begun. If this is not possible, the im dose/route should be used. Administration of routine booster doses of vaccine depends on exposure risk category as noted below. Preexposure immunization of immunosuppressed persons is not recommended.

Criteria for Preexposure Immunization

Risk category	Nature of risk	Typical populations	Preexposure regimen
Continuous	Virus present continuously, often in high concentrations; specific exposures likely to go unrecognized; bite, nonbite, or aerosol exposure	Rabies research lab workers* Rabies biologics production workers	Primary course; serologic testing every 6 months; booster vaccination if antibody titer is below acceptable level[†]
Frequent	Exposure usually episodic with source recognized, but exposure may also be unrecognized; bite, nonbite, or aerosol exposure possible	Rabies diagnostic lab workers,* spelunkers, veterinarians and staff, and animal control and wildlife workers in rabies-epizootic areas	Primary course; serologic testing every 2 years; booster vaccination if antibody titer is below acceptable level[†]

Table 3.10. (cont'd)

Criteria for Preexposure Immunization

Risk category	Nature of risk	Typical populations	Preexposure regimen
Infrequent (greater than population at large)	Exposure nearly always episodic with source recognized; bite or nonbite exposure	Veterinarians and animal control and wildlife workers in areas with low rabies rates; veterinary students Travelers visiting areas where rabies is enzootic and immediate access to appropriate medical care, including biologics, is limited	Primary course; no serologic testing or booster vaccination
Rare (population at large)	Exposure always episodic, with source recognized; bite or nonbite exposure	U.S. population at large, including individuals in rabies-epizootic areas	No preexposure immunization necessary

II. POSTEXPOSURE IMMUNIZATION. All postexposure treatment should begin with immediate thorough cleansing of all wounds with soap and water.

Persons not previously immunized: RIG, 20 IU/kg body weight, infiltrated at bite site (if possible), remainder im; 5 doses of HDCV, PCEC, or RVA, 1.0 mL im (i.e., deltoid area), 1 each on days 0, 3, 7, 14 and 28.

Persons previously immunized:

§ Two doses of HDCV, PCEC, or RVA. 1.0 mL, im (i.e., deltoid area), 1 each on days 0 and 3. RIG should not be administered.

* Judgment of relative risk and extra monitoring of vaccination status of laboratory workers is the responsibility of the laboratory supervisor (see U.S. Department of Health and Human Service's Biosafety in Microbiological and Biomedical Laboratories, 1984).

† Preexposure booster immunization consists of one dose of HDCV, PCEC, or RVA, 1.0 mL/dose, im (deltoid area) or HDCV, 0.1 mL id (deltoid). Minimum acceptable antibody level is complete virus neutralization at a 1:5 serum dilution by the rapid fluorescent focus inhibition test. A booster dose should be administered if titer falls below this level.

§ Preexposure immunization with HDCV, PCEC, or RVA; prior postexposure prophylaxis with HDCV, PCEC, or RVA; or persons previously immunized with any other type of rabies vaccine *and* a documented history of positive antibody response to the prior vaccination. Adapted from Health Information for International Travel, Centers for Disease Control.

IMMUNIZATIONS

- If the traveler will be taking chloroquine or mefloquine for malaria chemoprophylaxis, the 3-dose HCDV series must be completed before antimalarials are begun; if this is not possible, the im dose/route should be used.
- Administration of routine booster doses of vaccine depends on exposure risk category as noted below.
- Preexposure immunization of immunosuppressed persons is not recommended.

Indications: Long-term travelers to endemic areas especially children, those with outdoor occupations, adventure traveling to remote endemic areas; key considerations are duration and remoteness of trip and expected availability of postexposure treatment in the event of exposure; note that rabies immune globulin is often hard to obtain in many developing countries, which is a key rationale for preexposure vaccination (J Travel Med 1999;6:238)

Immunogenicity: 100% antibody formation

Booster: Often every 2 yr, but check antibody level every yr; if >30 IU, probably immune for long time; if <30 IU, will require regular boosting to keep level >0.5 IU; an alternative, more cost-effective approach: Boost all at year 1, check antibody level 2 wks later; if >30 IU, no further boosting needed for 10 yrs; if <30 IU, retest in 3 yr (Vaccine 2001;19:1416)

Side effects: Pain, erythema, itching 3–5%, mild systemic symptoms rarely; boosters, 6% type 1 or 3 rxn w repeat use HCDV; can substitute different vaccine in this event

Prevent:
- Travelers must understand need for 2 doses postexposure vaccine in event of bite despite use of preexposure regimen; however, rabies immune globulin will not be needed if preexposure prophylaxix (PEP) has been given
- If rabies exposure overseas, check w embassy re: reliable source of rx
- Note that equine rabies immune globulin is only type available in some countries, can cause serum sickness in 1%, anaphylaxis in 1/40,000

Table 3.11. Dosage and schedules for typhoid fever vaccination

Vaccination	Age	Dose/mode of administration	Number of doses	Interval between doses	Boosting interval (yr)
		Dose			
		Oral live-attenuated Ty21a vaccine			
Primary series	≥6 yr	1 capsule*	4	48 hr	5
		Vi capsular polysaccharide vaccine			
Primary series	≥2 yr	05 mL im	1	—	2
		Heat-phenol-inactivated parenteral vaccine			
Primary series	6 mo–10 yr	0.25 mL sc	2	≥4 wk	
	≥10 yr	0.50 mL sc	2	≥4 wk	3

* Administer with cool liquid no warmer than 37°C (98.6°F).

Table 3.12. Common adverse reactions to typhoid fever vaccines

Vaccine	Fever (%)	Headache (%)	Local reactions
		Reactions	
Ty21a*	0–5	0–5	Not applicable
ViCPS	0–1	1.5–3	Erythema or induration ≥ cm: 7%
Parenteral inactivated	6.7–24	9–10	Severe local pailn or swelling: 3–35%

* The side effects of Ty21a are rare and mainly consist of abdominal discomfort, nausea, vomiting, and rash or urticaria.
Adapted from Health Information for International Travel, Centers for Disease Control.

3.12 TYPHOID VACCINE

Arch Intern Med 1998;158:663; BMJ 1998;316:110

Disease: Fever, often w complications, caused by *Salmonella typhi*; estimated 30 million cases annually, w 500,000 deaths; via contaminated food and water (see 16.51)

Indications: Travelers going outside usual tourist routes in So America, Africa, Asia; risk varies from 1–800/million travelers to developing countries; consider in all travelers to Indian subcontinent

Vaccine: Three licensed vaccines: oral live attenuated vaccine (Vivotif), strain Ty21a, Vi a capsular polysaccharide vaccine (V, CPS), parenteral vaccine (Typhim V); heat phenol inactivated vaccine (rarely used now due to side effects); see Tables 3.11 and 3.12. New S. typhi Vi conjugate vaccine (Vi-rEPA) safe and effective (90% efficacy) in children age 2–5 yr (Nejm 2001;344:1263)

Efficacy: 70–80% (recent reports of failures in Dutch tourists; J Trav Med 2000;7:19); note decr immunogenicity of live vaccine w concomitant antibiotic or mefloquine use

Boosters: Every 5 yr for Ty21 A, 2–3 yr for Typhim V

Side effects: See Table 3.12; avoid antibiotics with oral vaccine

Contraindications: Ty21a not to be used in immunocompromised pts or children <2 yr; avoid in pregnancy; allergic rxns to any formulation

3.13 TETANUS/DIPHTHERIA VACCINE

Mmwr 2000;49:1

Disease: Tetanus—toxin associated after trauma (skin puncture, etc.) Diphtheria—severe toxin-mediated pharyngitis (see 16.45)

Indications: Routine childhood vaccine—DPT (tetanus, diphtheria, pertussis); now DtaP w acellular pertussis (only need Td in adults); because of diphtheria outbreaks in Eastern Europe and elsewhere, travelers need Td up to date

Vaccine: 4 vaccines containing diptheria/tetanus toxoids and acellular pertussis now available; primary series in 4–5 doses

Efficacy: >99%

Booster: Tetanus/diptheria every 10 yr

Side effects: Local reaction common with tenderness, erythema, induration

Contraindications: Serious rxn to prior vaccination; use same brand for all pediatric doses of DTaP

3.14 POLIO VACCINE

Mmwr 1999;48:416; Pediatrics 1997;99:300

Disease: Acute enteroviral infection with gastroenteritis followed by possible paralytic CNS disease—fecal/oral transmission (see 20.14)

Indications: Polio transmission occurs in developing countries of Africa, Asia, Eastern Europe, and the Middle East, though risk is decreasing w eradication campaign; No and So America considered polio free, but outbreak in Haiti/Dominican Republic in 2000 w vaccine-associated strain; global eradication program is well underway, but adult travelers to endemic areas need a booster after primary series

Vaccine: Routine childhood vaccine: primary series is 3 doses of either oral live attenuated (OPV) or inactivated polio vaccine (eIPV); IPV now recommended for all, booster needed 1 time only in travelers who have received the primary series; OPV no longer available in the U.S.

Efficacy: eIPV: 97–100% after 2 doses

Side effects: Minor local reaction, pain and erythema after IPV, possibility of vaccine-associated paralytic polio (VAPP) after OPV (risk <1/million)

Contraindication (eIPV): Allergy to neomycin, polymyxin B

3.15 LYME DISEASE VACCINE

Mmwr 1999;48:7

Disease: Tick-borne spirochetal zoonosis of temperate zones of North America and Eurasia

Indications: Individuals (age 15–70) w frequent or prolonged exposure to deer-tick-infested habitats in endemic areas of the U.S./Canada; note that current vaccine may not be effective against European strains of *B. burgdorferi* (see 16.24)

Vaccine: Recombinant *B. burgdorferi* lipidated outer surface protein A (Osp A) as immunogen (Lymerix SKB); given im 0.5 mL in 3 doses; FDA approved for 0, 1, 12 mo schedule, but 0, 1, 2, or 6 mo schedule also appears effective (CID 1999;28:1260)

IMMUNIZATIONS

Immunogenicity/efficacy: 76% efficacy after 3 doses (100% effective in preventing asymptomatic seroconversion); titers of 1200 ELISA units/mL correlates w protection; extrapolation of these results and fall in antibody levels suggests need for booster every 1–2 yr

Booster: See above; interval not determined

Side effects: Soreness at injection site (20%); myalgias, fever, chills (<3%)

Contraindication: Pregnancy, immunocompromised; active treatment unresponsive Lyme arthritis; not approved for pediatric use

3.16 TICK-BORNE ENCEPHALITIS VACCINE (not available in U.S.)

CID 1999;28:882

Disease: Arboviral encephalitis (see 20.2) transmitted by *Ixodes* ticks ("sheep ticks") in Eurasia (see Fig. 3.6); also by unpasteurized milk

Indications: For travelers who anticipate extensive exposure to ticks in rural areas endemic for tick-borne encephalitis (ie, persons planning prolonged hiking trips or field biologists etc.); risk is highly focal; consult local authorities to assess

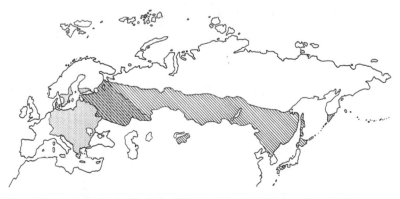

Figure 3.6. Geographic distribution of Western (dots) and Eastern (lines) of the tick-borne encephalitis virus. (Reproduced with permission from CID 1999;28:883.)

Vaccine:
1. Formaldelhyde inactivated purified whole virus (FSME-Immune; Immune AG-Austria)
2. Similar inactivated purified whole virus (Encepur; FSME vaccine Behring)
3. Russian vaccine (similar) (Academy of Medical Sciences, Moscow)

For 1 and 2, give 3 doses; 2 approved for accelerated schedule (0, 7, 21 d)

Efficacy: Estimated at 90–95% after 3 doses

Booster: Every 3–5 yr (boost at 12–18 mo after accelerated schedule)

Side effects: Local inflammation at injection site; flu-like reactions; allergic rxns

Contraindications: Incr risk of anaphylaxis in pts prone to allergic rxn; do not give during acute infections

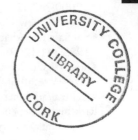

4 Prevention of Malaria (See also 18.25)

Inf Dis Clin N Am 1998;12:267; Arch IM 2000;160:2505

Key elements:
- Assessment of risk (for current info see CDC Resources below)
- Antimosquito measures
- Consideration of chemoprophylaxis options
- Traveler educaton re: malaria sx/si

Assessment of risk: >1500 cases/yr/U.S.; 30,000 cases/yr in travelers from industrialized countries to developing countries; imported falciparum malaria mortality overall is 0.6–3.7% (Ann IM 1990;113:326); falciparum malaria, mostly from chloroquine resistant areas, incr in U.S./Canadian travelers, accounts for 1/3 imported cases; marked variation in risk depends on itinerary, season, activity (ie, night-time mosquito exposure), elevation (<2000 m)

Geographic risk: Estimate per month per unprotected traveler (Nejm 2000;342:1716)
- Oceania/New Guinea: up to 20% in some areas
- SubSaharan Africa: 2%; majority of cases are *P. falciparum* (Lancet 1993;341:1299)
- South Asia: 0.1–0.01%, mostly *P. vivax* (Trans Roy Soc Trop Med Hyg 1996;90:680)
- Central/So America: 0.01%

Risk highly dependent on activity (= degree of mosquito exposure); accounts in part for high risk in African travelers, most of whom visit game parks vs urban Asian travelers; attack rates reached 50% in tourists on African river raft trip (CID 1999;337:1140); see CDC resources (Health Information for Intl Travel, voice info 888-232-3228; fax 888-232-3299; or internet <http.//www.cdc.gov/travel/index.htm>); See malaria map, Fig. 4.1

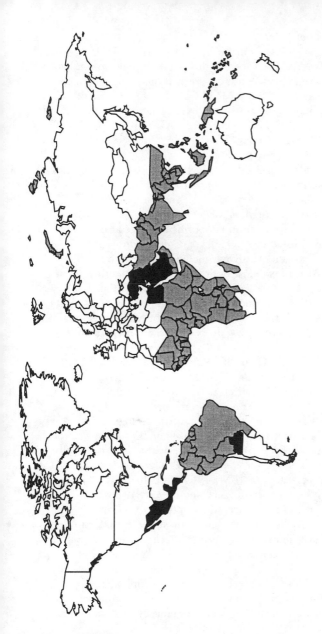

Figure 4.1. Distribution of malaria and chloroquine-resistant *Plasmodium falciparum*. (Reproduced from Health Information for International Travel, CDC.)

● Chloroquine-resistant *P. falciparum*

● Chloroquine-sensitive malaria

MALARIA

Antimosquito measures:

DEET-containing repellants on skin (usually 30–35% DEET for 4 hr protection effective) (see 7.5 re arthropod bite prevention); avoid evening/night-time bites w use of screened quarters or permethrin treated bed nets (Am J Trop Med Hyg 1990;43:11); use of pyrethroid containing insect sprays in sleeping areas may also help

USE OF CHEMOPROPHYLAXIS DOES NOT OBVIATE NEED FOR THESE MEASURES

Chemoprophylaxis of malaria:

Risk/benefit depends on individual travel plans (ie, determine if travel involves exposure to malaria, if choloroquine-resistant *P. falciparum* malaria is present, whether there are medical contraindications for use of a particular agent); CDC resources listed above give current country specific info; see also travel advice resources listed in Appendix 1. *Consideration* of chemoprophylaxis should always include travelers to urban/rural SubSaharan Africa (exc most of So Africa), Oceania (incl Papua New Guinea, Irian Jaya, Vanuatu), Haiti, India, Bangladesh, Pakistan, Nepal (Terai region), evening/night exposure in rural areas of SE Asia, C and So America, parts of Mexico, Dominican Republic, No Africa (Inf Dis Clin NA 1998;12:267); options (see Table 4.1)

FOR AREAS OF CHLOROQUINE SENSITIVE *P. FALCIPARUM* ONLY (ie, Haiti, Dominican Republic, Central America w of Panama Canal Zone, Egypt, most countries of Middle East): Chloroquine phosphate (Aralen) 300 mg base (500 mg salt) po once/wk; start 1–2 wk prior to travel, q wk during, and for 4 wk after leaving malarious areas; may cause mild GI upset, dizzyness, headache, blurred vision, pruritus, exacerbate psoriasis; usually well-tolerated (and w/o risk retinopathy) in prophylaxis doses; safe in pregnancy—category C. (BMJ 1985;290:1466)

Long-term users (ie, 5 yr or 100 gms) should have regular ophthalmologic exams; contraindic in pts w preexisting retinopathy, CNS disorders; concomitant use w HCDV id rabies vaccine may decr immune response to vaccine (use im dosing of HCDV in this instance); pediatric dose is 5 mg/kg/wk; overall efficacy >90%

FOR OTHER AREAS (Except Thai borders w Cambodia, Myanmar): Can use mefloquine, doxycycline, atovaquone/proguanil, primaquine; all w protective efficacy vs *P. falciparum*

Table 4.1. Drugs used in the prophylaxis of malaria

Drug	Usage	Adult dose	Pediatric dose	Comments
Mefloquine (Lariam)	In areas with chloroquine-resistant *Plasmodium falciparum*	228 mg base (250 mg salt) orally, once/wk	<15 kg: 4.6 mg/kg base (5 mg/kg [salt]) once/wk 15–19 kg: 1/4 tab/wk 20–30 kg: 1/2 tab/wk 31–45 kg: 3/4 tab/wk >45 kg: 1 tab/wk	Contraindicated in persons allergic to mefloquine. Not recommended for persons with epilepsy and other seizure disorders; with severe psychiatric disorders; or with cardiac conduction abnormalities.
Doxycycline	An alternative to mefloquine	100 mg orally, once/d	>8 yr of age: 2 mg/kg of body weight orally/d up to adult dose of 100 mg/d	Contraindicated in children <8 yr of age, pregnant women, and lactating women.
Chloroquine phosphate (Aralen)	In areas with chloroquine-sensitive *Plasmodium falciparum*	300 mg base (500 mg salt) orally, once/wk	5 mg/kg base (8.3 mg/kg [salt]) orally, once/wk, up to maximum adult dose of 300 mg base	
Hydroxy-chloroquine sulfate (Plaquenil)	An alternative to chloroquine	310 mg base (400 mg salt) orally, once/wk	5 mg/kg base (6.5 mg/kg [salt]) orally, once/wk, up to maximum adult dose of 310 mg base	
Chloroquine + proguanil	A less effective alternative for use in Africa, only if mefloquine or doxycycline cannot be used	Weekly chloroquine dose as above, plus daily proguanil dose 200 mg orally, once/d	Weekly chloroquine dose as above, plus <2 yr: 50 mg/d 2–6 yr: 100 mg/d 7–10 yr: 150 mg/d >10 yr: 200 mg/d	Proguanil is not sold in the U.S., but is widely available in Canada, Europe, and many African countries.
Atovaquone + proguanil (Malarone)	Alternative mefloquine	250 mg atovaquone/ 100 mg proguanil one tab/d	62.5 mg atovaquone/25 mg proguanil; dose based on weight	Can start 1 day before exposure, discontinue 7 days after. Take with food.

Adapted from Health Information for International Travel, Centers for Disease Control.

MALARIA

of >90% in nonimmune travelers; also effective against other malaria species

- Mefloquine: dosage is 250 mg (228 mg base) q wk, starting 2–3 wk prior to trip, q wk during exposure, and 4 wk after; (altern: loading dose of one tab/d × 3 d may be used during wk before travel); ped dose noted in Table 4.1; side effects include ha, insomnia, irritability, weakness, diarrhea; but intolerable in <5% (BMJ 1996;313:525)

Severe neuropsych rxns in 1/13,000 (JID 1996;173:1506); rare prolonged QT interval, toxic epidermal necrolysis (Lancet 1997;349:101); no adverse effect on performance of airplane pilots (Am J Trop Med Hyg 1997;56:235); well-tolerated long-term in Peace Corps users (Lancet 1993;341:848); contraindic in pts w preexisting neuropsych disease (esp epilepsy), allergy to quinines; note potential for interaction w quinine, w antiarrhythmic medications; appears safe for concomitant use w β-blockers, but avoid w pts w cardiac conduction abnormalities; category C for pregnancy, w evidence of safety after first trimester (JID 1994;169:595); w/o evidence of danger in first trimester by post-marketing surveillance (Am J Trop Med Hyg 1998;58:17), but should avoid; note that mefloquine may persist in human for 3 mo after use; overall efficacy in malaria prevention > 90% w *P. falciparum* as noted, exc rare foci (ie, Thai border), and *P. vivax* in some areas

- Doxycyline: altern to mefloquine, requires daily use, 100 mg/d, started 1–2 d prior to trip, qd during trip, 4 wk after (Ann IM 1994;120:294); side effects incl diarrhea, nausea, photosensitivity, monilial vaginitis; contraindic in pregnancy, in children <8 yo, h/o allergy to tetracyclines; use sunscreen if on doxycycline w sun exposure

- Atovaquone/proguanil: approved by FDA in U.S. in 2000 for prophylaxis/rx malaria; dose for adults is one tab (250 mg atov/100 mg prog) qd, starting 1–2 d before trip, continuing qd during exposure, and 7 d after leaving malarious area; pediatric approval for children >11 kg (see 9.3); take w food as decr bioavail w/o fat; also antacids, tetracyclines may decr absorption. Side effects incl abd pain, headache, but fewer GI side effects than choroquine/proguanil (Lancet 2000;356:1888); do not administer w rifampin, metoclopramide; not approved for use in pregnancy; effective causal prophylaxis (ie, kills preerythrocytic stages of *P.*

Table 4.2. Presumptive treatment of malaria

Drug	Adult dose	Pediatric dosage	Comment
Pyrimethamine-sulfadoxine (Fansidar). Self-treatment drug to be used if professional medical care is not available within 24 hours. *Seek medical care immediately after self-treatment!*	3 tablets (75 mg pyrimethamine and 1,500 mg sulfadoxine), orally as a single dose	5–10 kg: 1/2 tablet 11–20 kg: 1 tablet 21–30 kg: 1 1/2 tablets 31–45 kg: 2 tablets >45 kg: 3 tablets	Contraindicated in persons with sulfa allergy

Note: Do not rely on this regimen for returning travelers (see 18.25)
Adapted from Health Information for International Travel, Centers for Disease Control.

falciparum malaria, permits short course rx after exposure (Lancet 2000;356:1864)
- Primaquine: similar efficacy to regimens noted above (Ann IM 1998;129:241); dose 0.5 mg base/kg/d (30 mg/d for most adults >70 kg), starting 1–2 d before trip, continuing during trip and 1–7 d after; side effects incl GI upset; contraindic w G6PD defic; rare methemoglob; effective causal prophylaxis; may have role in areas w high risk of *P. vivax* as relapse of liver parasite infx is prevented (CID 1999;29:1592); not approved in pregnancy

FOR THAI-KAMPUCHEA/MYANMAR BORDER AREAS: Multiresistant *P. falciparum* predominates; prophylaxis w doxycycline or atovaquone/proguanil preferred

FOR TRAVELERS WITH INTENSE P. VIVAX/OVALE EXPOSURE: Relapse of malaria may occur in travelers infected w *P. vivax/ovale* malaria due to reemergence into blood of primary or secondary liver stages following suppression w chloroquine, mefloquine, doxycycline, atovaquone/proguanil; primaquine given during the last 2 wk of chemoprophylaxis (terminal prophylaxis) is effective in preventing these relapses; dose 0.5 mg/kg/d × 14 d; due to appearance of primaquine-resistant strains of *P. vivax* in some areas of SE Asia, Oceania, Somalia, some experts recommend using higher dose (30 mg/d) in these returning travelers

Self-treatment of malaria in travelers: Controversial; for travelers unable to take effective prophylactic regimens but who are at substantial malaria risk in areas w/o health care access; CDC rec self-treatment w pyrimethamine/sulfadoxine (Fansidar-3 tablets single dose) as an option for rx high fever until transport to a medical facility (see Table 4.2). Another option for self-treatment is Malorone (adult Rx dose: 4 tabs daily for 3d). Contact CDC for updated geographic recommendations.

Traveler education regarding malaria: Travelers to malarious areas should be informed that all of the preventive measures noted above may fail; any febrile illness (even w predom resp or GI sx) occurring in the few months after return merits prompt attention and consideration of malaria; pamphlets from CDC and others are available for travelers

5 Prevention of Food- and Waterborne Disease

Textbook of Travel Medicine and Health, Hamilton, Ontario, B.C. Decker, 1997; ch 12.2

Key Elements:
- Recognition of risks/foods to avoid
- Water disinfection
- Chemoprophylaxis for traveler's diarrhea
- Self-treatment of traveler's diarrhea
- Vaccination

RECOGNITION OF RISKS

Due to sanitary lapses in food handling and water treatment, travelers from developed countries to developing countries are at high risk for a variety of enteric infections grouped under the sobriquet of "traveler's diarrhea" (see 16.47). In addition to self-limited diarrhea, more serious infections may follow exposure to contaminated food or water. Examples include viral hepatitis (A, E), typhoid/paratyphoid fever, leptospirosis, and a variety of bacterial, parasitic, viral infections. Particular foods present specific risks (ie, unpasteurized milk can cause listeriosis, brucellosis, rat bite fever, yersinia). Raw or undercooked meats risk brucellosis, toxoplasmosis, salmonella, trichinosis (pork); shellfish concentrate particulate matter from seawater, and therefore are vehicles for enteric infections in contaminated waters (ie, hep A, typhoid, *Vibrio* infections) and can be the source of toxin-related disease (ie, paralytic shellfish poisoning), partic in regions where shellfish are not monitored for safety. Raw fish or other invertebrates are the source of parasitic diseases (ie, anasakiasis, etc.) and toxin-related diseases such as scombroid, ciguaterra poisoning, tetrodotoxin. Aquatic plants (ie, watercress, etc.), esp in Asia, may be the source for parasitic diseases such as clonorchiasis. Unwashed (or washed in untreated water) fruits and vegetables often are contaminated w fecal bacteria/parasites due to the use of human and animal feces as fertilizer. Foods left standing in hot environments may provide nutrients for various bacterial pathogens, incl toxin producing strains of *S. aureus*, *Bacillus cereus*, *Clostridium perfringens*, etc.

General advice re: safe foods:
- "Boil it, cook it, peel it, or forget it"
- Foods thoroughly cooked at 160°F kill most bacteria (Arch IM 1988;148:2261); these will be "too hot to eat" when first served
- "Dry" foods, such as breads, are usually safe, as are packaged foods
- raw or undercooked seafood (ie, ceviche, sashimi) is risky in many areas
- salads should be carefully washed in treated water; often not done
- dairy products should be pasteurized
- fruits should be peeled; beware watermelons, etc., injected to incr wght
- location/culinary practices important to minimize cross-contamination (ie, avoid street vendors or cooking sites w flies and w/o refrigeration)

WATER DISINFECTION

Water is potential source of enteric disease, esp parasitic disease such as *Giardia, Cryptosporidium*, and viral diseases (hep A, hep E). Tap water is often unsafe in developing countries, as are unsealed "pure" water bottles. Ice cubes carry viable pathogens (Jama 1985;253:3141). Safe water is disinfected by boiling or other treatment methods. Approved methods of water disinfection incl:
1. Boiling (to a rolling boil for 1 min); at >6500 ft (2 km), boil for 3 min
2. Chemical treatment (for short-term, wk use); iodoine preferred over chlorine: tincture of iodine (see Table 5.1): use tetraglycine hydroperiodide tablets (double # if cloudy water; incr contact time

Table 5.1. Treatment of water with tincture of iodine

Tincture of iodine (from medicine chest or first aid kit)	Drops* to be added per quart or liter	
	Clear water	Cold or cloudy water[†]
2%	5	10

* 1 drop = 0.05 mL. Let stand for 30 minutes before water is safe to use.
[†] Very turbid or very cold water may require prolonged contact time; let stand up to several hours prior to use, if possible. To ensure that *Cryptosporidium* is killed, water must stand for 15 hours before drinking.
Adapted from Health Information for International Travel, Centers for Disease Control.

for very cold water; note shelf life of product once opened; for short-term (wks) use only

3. Water filters: many types that remove parasites/bacteria, but reliability vs viruses is less certain; reverse osmosis or iodine resin filters most likely to remove all microorganisms, but depend on proper use; in developing countries, may not want to rely on filter exclusivley (Wilderness Env Med 2000;11:1); additional information re: filters passing NSF testing: call 1-800-673-8010 or write to NSF 3475 Plymouth Rd, PO Box 130140, Ann Arbor MI 48113-0140

CHEMOPROPHYLAXIS OF TRAVELER'S DIARRHEA

Generally not recommended; bismuth subsalicyate (2 oz qid or 2 tabs qid) decr incidence of TD by 60% (Nejm 1993;328:1821) but is burdensome, turns stools black but safe; antimicrobial prophylaxis w antibiotics causes minor se in 3%, serious se in 0.01%; effective in 50–90%, but varies w geography/season/etc.; may be chosen for well-informed travelers w higher risk from enteric infx (ie, pts w HIV, other immunosuppression, etc.); new lactobacillus preparation (ie, lactobacillus gg) may prove helpful; see 16.47 for more information.

SELF-TREATMENT OF TRAVELER'S DIARRHEA

Mild sx may be palliated w bismuth subsalicyate, or antimotility agents such as loperamide, which traveler can obtain OTC; prescription of short courses of antibiotics (see 16.47) is highly effective for most TD but pts need to be made aware (preferably w written instruction) of how and when to use them, se, potential drug interactions: Usual course is 1–3 d po antibiotic, except in event of traveler in remote area w dysenteric sx, where 5–7 d may be taken. In general, travelers should be counseled to seek medical help for severe, persistent sx rather than rely on empiric self-treatment

VACCINATIONS

Effective vaccines for TD not yet available, but under study; vaccinations against hepatitis A, typhoid (and in some limited circumstancs, cholera) may be advised as outlined in 3.5 and 3.12.

6 Prevention of Accidents and Injuries

Textbook of Travel Medicine and Health, B.C. Decker, 1997;21:1

Key Elements:
- Epidemiology of accidents and injuries (see Fig. 6.1)
- Contributing causes and prevention of motor vehicle accidents
- Considerations in particular groups of travelers

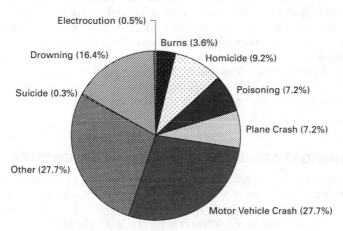

Figure 6.1. Injury death of American travelers, unintentional and intentional.

EPIDEMIOLOGY

Accidental injuries cause 20–25% of travel related deaths overall (Ann Emerg Med 1991;44:622; Int J Epidem 1991;19:225; J Travel Med 2000;7:227). Up to 70% in younger groups of travelers, such as Peace Corps (Jama 1985;254:1326); motor vehicle accidents account for 25–60% of these deaths (Jama 1985;254:1326; also Am J Trop Med Hyg 1992;46:686). Drownings are next most common (12–18%), followed by homicide, suicide, falls, animal attacks, etc. Mortality overall not demonstrably different than domestic for same age group, but risk varies markedly between countries and travel goups. Injuries account for only 2% of morbidity (JID 1987;156:84).

CONTRIBUTING CAUSES AND PREVENTION OF MOTOR VEHICLE ACCIDENTS

Car/motorcycle accidents most important; in Peace Corps, motorcycles involved in 1/3 of all crashes, caused 12% of mortality. (Jama 1985;254:1326). Review of motor vehicle deaths among missionaries to Africa revealed frequent lack of seatbelts or their use, riding in nonpassenger areas (ie, back of open truck, etc.), poor vehicle/ road maintenance (Travel Med 1989; 67). Suggested targets for intervention include: emphasis on use of seatbelts; avoidance of night-time driving; careful selection of vehicles/drivers.

CONSIDERATIONS FOR PARTICULAR GROUPS

Trekkers represent a potentially high-risk group; one study in 1980s revealed death rate of 15 per 100,000 trekking pernits, w helicopter rescue in 75 per 100,000. Trauma accounted for 11 deaths, illness for 8, and acute mountain sickness for 3 (Jama 1989;261:1017).

7 Prevention of Environmental Illnesses

7.1 ALTITUDE ILLNESS

Mayo Clin Proc 1998;73:988; Nejm 2001;345:107

Cause: Ambient Po_2 decr w incr altitude, esp >8500 ft

Epidem: Risk incr w altitude and rapidity of ascent; 20% skiers at high altitude resorts are affected w acute mountain sickness (Ann IM 1993;118:587); risk incr w residence at <3000 ft, w age <60, or w underlying lung problems, or prior hx altitude illness; serious conditions (ie, high alt pulm edema; HAPE) are much rarer in similar tourists (0.01%); high altitude cerebral edema (HACE) also rare, affects 2–3% of trekkers at >18,000 ft

Risk for travelers: Frequent problem w rapid ascents (esp flights) to high altitude destinations (>8000 ft); serious complications of HAPE or HACE are of concern to travelers to very high altitude (>11,000 ft); onset of HAPE is often second night after steep ascent; stable CAD or CHF not a risk at moderate altitude (Am J Med 2000;109;450); in pregnancy, limit alt to 12,000 ft, and avoid in complicated pregnancies; sickle cell crises can be provoked at >1500 m

Pathophys:
- Acute mt sickness (AMS): hypoxia causes incr ventilation w respiratory alkalosis
- HAPE: incr pulmonary artery pressure and vascular permeability (inflammatory mediators present in bronchoalveolar lavage; Jama 1986;256:63)
- HACE: ? vasogenic (reversible white matter edema on MRI; Jama 1998;280:1920)

57

Sx:

- Acute mountain sickness: headache, nausea, fatigue, dizziness, anorexia, insomnia, dyspnea; sx typically developed w/in 6–10 h of ascent, persist for 1–3 d after ascent
- HAPE: progressive DOE to dyspnea at rest, dry cough, weakness, chest tightness
- HACE: Severe ha, loss of balance, confusion, drowsiness

Si:

- AMS: none, except occas peripheral edema, nocturnal periodic breathing (w/o other sx)
- HAPE: tachycardia, tachypnea, rales, pink sputum, cyanosis, low grade fever
- HACE: altered mental state, papilledema, ataxia, sometimes CN palsies; note that retinal hemorrhages may occur at >15,000 ft w/o HACE

Crs:

- AMS resolves w acclimatization over several days; HAPE and HACE become life-threatening unless rapid descent

Rx:

- AMS: Slow or stop ascent; acetazolamide 125–250 mg bid (Ann IM 1992;116:461); dexamethasone also effective (Nejm 1989;321:1707)
- HAPE: immediate descent of 500–1000 m (or Gamov hyperbaric bag); keep warm; nifedipine 10 mg orally; then 30 mg of extended release formulation po q 12–24 h (Nejm 1991;325:1284); oxygen (4–6 L/min or hyperbaric); add dexamethasone if neurologic deterioration
- HACE: immediate descent of 500–1000 m; dexamethasone 4–10 mg iv followed by 4 mg (po or iv) q 6 h; high flow O_2 or portable hyperbaric chamber

Prevent:

- AMS: slow ascent (<500 m/d); avoid abrupt ascents to >3000 m (ie, spend 1–2 d at intermediate altitude; do not raise sleep altitude by >1000 ft /d); acetazolamide 24 h before ascent and for 2–3 d after (note recommended doses vary from 125 mg bid to 250 mg tid; recent meta-analysis suggests higher dose; BMJ 2000;321:267) but side effects more frequent

Note: do not use acetazoleamide if sulfa allergic; side effects include parethesias, metallic taste, polyuria; dexamethasone (8–16 mg/d) also effective (Nejm 1984;310:683)

- HAPE: slow ascent; prophylactic nifedipine (20 mg–30 mg extended release q 12 h) may have utility in those at high risk (Nejm 1991;325:1284), esp w prior h/o HAPE

7.2 HEAT ILLNESS

Nejm 1993;329:483

Cause: Environmental heat exposure (ie, temp >95°F w high humidity) combined w vigorous actvity or lack of acclimatization; wet bulb thermometer best predicts environmental risk

Epidem: Predisposing conditions include youth (children more prone to heat injury), medications that decrease sweating (ie, phenothiazines, anticholinergics) or diuretics, or sympathomimetics

Heat cramps or edema, or heat exhaustion are not uncommon; heat stroke is rare, follows extreme efforts w/o rest; every year, hundreds of deaths occur during the hajj

Risk for travelers: Associated w vigorous exertion (ie, athletics, treks, etc.) w/o prior acclimatization; minor heat illness is common; heat stroke extremely rare

Pathophys: Inability to adequately lose body heat due to decr sweating (high humidity, dehydration, etc). Acclimatization involves plasma volume incr; takes 10–14 d

Sx:
- Heat cramps—pain in lower extremity muscles (esp calves), usually in athletes
- Heat syncope—lightheadedness, often after prolonged standing, w syncope due to venous pooling w vasodilation
- Heat exhaustion—lightheadedness, fatigue, nausea, thirst, myalgias
- Heat stroke—confusion, extreme weakness

Si:
- Heat exhaustion—tachycardia, may have incr temp, orthostatic hypotension
- Heat stroke—altered mental state, hyperthermia, often no sweating

Crs: Heat stroke is a medical emergency (failure of thermoregulation); potentially fatal

Rx:
- Heat cramps—rest, oral rehydration solution
- Heat syncope—rest, shade, 1 L oral fluids
- Heat exhaustion—rest in shade, oral rehydration
- Heat stroke—rapid cooling (ice packs, wet w fanning to facilitate evaporation), NPO, iv fluids (1–2 L normal saline)

Prevent: Acclimatize before vigorous physical exercise when possible; plan adequate hydration for activities (500 mL water prior to exercise, w additional 300 mL q 20 min)

7.3 SUNBURN AND OTHER LIGHT REACTIONS

Lamberg; *Little Black Book Dermatol*; Blackwell Science, 2000

Cause: Due to excessive exposure to solar radiation; UVB (290–320 nm) esp, but also UVA, plus external or systemic photosensitizer

Epidem: Common in individuals experiencing incr exposure to sunlight; associated w excessive mid-day exposure, but esp w sun exposure near water, snow, or at high altitude; susceptibility incr w decr genetic ability to synthesize melanin

Risk for travelers: High for susceptible travelers, esp for those w regular outdoor activities near water or snow; photosensitive and phototoxic rxns incr by some frequently used medicines (ie, sulfa or tetracycline and some flourquinolone antibiotics or chloroquine); polymorphic light eruption (PMLE) common in winter visitors from northern areas to tropics; sun induced contact dermatitis may occur w contact w limes, other plants, esp in tropics

Time of onset:
- W/in minutes of exposure: solar urticaria
- W/in 48 hr of exposure: sunburn, phototoxic and photoallergic rxns, polymorphic light eruption, solar urticaria, SLE-assoc
- Weeks to months: some photoallergic drug rxns, SLE-assoc, porphyrias, etc.

Sx: Sunburn—pain, redness, tenderness
Phototoxic/allergic rxn—itching may predominate

Si: Sunburn—erythema (w blister in severe rxn) on sun-exposed areas
Solar urticaria—transient (1–2 h) hives
PMLE—nodules, uriticaria, scaly dermatitis restricted to sun-exposed areas
Phototoxic—exaggerated sunburn; sometimes persistent erythema w netted pattern
Photoallergic—dermatitis on sun-exposed areas
Phytophoto contact dermatitis—striated vesicular or bullous rxns may follow contact w some plants

Crs: Resolution w/in days w avoidance of sun, except for photoallergic rxns, PMLE, or systemic dermatologic diseases

Rx: Sunburn—ASA or other NSAID for pain relief; soothe severely affected areas w 20 min colloidal oatmeal bath (1/2 cup Aveeno oatmeal to bath); no benefit from topical or systemic steroids; PMLE—steroids (topical and systemic) may be beneficial

Prevent: When possible: use of protective clothing, avoidance of sun between 10 AM to 3 PM; Note high level sun exposure even on cloudy days

Sunscreens: Choices depends on expected exposure and type of rxn hx; ie, mild to moderate sunburn, PABA only containing sunscreens block UVB, but not UVA; benzophenone, anthranilate and other "broad spectrum" sunscreens provide some UVA protection as well, important in prevent of PMLE, drug-induced light eruptions, solar urticaria; for at risk travelers w intense exposure (ie, climbers, water sports enthusiasts, etc, opaque sunblockers helpful on uncovered areas; ie, titanium oxide or zinc oxide to nose, etc.)

Note that SPF of product indicates multiple of prolongation of time to sunburn; an SPF 15 means that if sun exposure likely to cause sunburn in 30 min w/o screen, addition of screen will prolong protection to 7.5 h; for shorter exposure, no benefit in SPF 30 over SPF 15; sunscreens should be applied 1–2 h before exposure, and reapplied after swimming or sweating

Rare allergic contact rxn to sunscreens may occur

Medication: Be aware of sun-sensitizing medications; see Table 7.1; take special precautions if applicable

Table 7.1. Sun-Sensitizing Medications

Antibiotics
Ciprofloxacin
Griseofulvin
Sulfa drugs
Tetracyclines

Anticancer Drugs
Actinomycin
Dacarbazine
Doxorubicin
5-FU

Antihistamines
Astemizole
Brompheniramine
Carbinoxamine
Cetirizine
Chlorpheniramine
Cyproheptadine
Diphenhydramine
Loratadine
Terfenadine

Antihypertensives
Captopril

Diuretics
Amiloride
Furosemide
Metolazone
Quinethazone
Thiazides

Hydroxyurea
MTX
Procarbazine
Vinblastine

Antidepressants/Antipsychotics
"Amines"
Amoxapine
Doxepin
Isocarboxazid
Tricyclic antidepressants
Triptylines

Hormones
Estrogens
Progestogens

Hypoglycemics
Acetohexamide
Chlorpropamide
Glipizide
Glyburide
Tolazamide
Tolbutamide

NSAIDs
Diclofenac
Indomethacin
Naproxen
Phenylbutazone
Profens
Piroxicam
Sulindac

Adapted from Health Information for International Travel, Centers for Disease Control.

7.4 COLD EXPOSURE AND INJURIES

Postgrad Med 1999;105:72

Cause: Body cannot conserve heat or prevent heat loss

Epidem: Hypothermia associated w outdoor exposure in cold climates, but may occur in temperate climates w water immersion or nocturnal exposure (esp in desert areas) w/o adequate protection, esp w predisposing factors (ie, alcohol or sedative intoxication); incr risk in children (higher surface to body ratio) and elderly (decr vasoconstrictive response, ability to shiver)

Risk for travelers: Severe injury (hypothermia) rare, usually due to prolonged exposure at high altitude or water immersion w/o facilities for rewarming (ie, canoe/kayak/sailing trips in cold waters); minor illness (ie, frostnip or mild frostbite) common in winter outdoor enthusiasts

Pathophys: Heat loss by radiation (esp from unprotected head), evaporation/respiration (20–30%), conduction/convection; wet clothing incr heat loss 5×, water immersion up to 25×

Shivering incr BMR 5×; responses to heat loss include peripheral vasoconstriction; main effects drop in core temp are CNS and cardiovascular; at core temp 35°C, CNS rxns slowed, tachycardia followed by bradycardia; at core temp 32.2°C (90°F), CNS flow decr w mental status change, myocardial irritablility develops

Sx:

- Hypothermia: mild (T 32–35°C), tachycardia, shivering, incoordination, fatigue, dizziness; moderate (30–32°C) lethargy, confusion; severe (<30°C) severe disorientation, coma
- Frostnip/frostbite: pale or blue discolored area of skin, decr sensation (usually distal extremity or exposed area of face); frostbite leads to throbbing pain 48–72 hr after injury w persistent tingling
- Trenchfoot (immersion foot): swollen numb foot (follows prolonged exp of foot to wet cold)
- Chilblain (pernio): small painful eruption over exposed areas (follows prolonged exp to dry cold)

ENVIRONMENTAL

Si:

- Hypothermia: decr core temp (NOT shell temp; measure w rectal or esophageal probe); mental status changes, cardiac arrhythmias; dysarthria, tachypnea, tachycardia, hyperreflexia (mild); absence of shivering, stupor, pupillary dilatation, decr respiration, bp, reflexes w mod/severe
- Frostbite: vesicles/bullae form at 6–24 hr; black eschar may form at 9–15 d; lack of sensation over affected areas

Rx:

- Hypothermia: shelter pt, cover (aluminized body cover = space blanket), remove wet clothes; provide passive rewarming w dry blanket or dry clothing; careful transport to hospital (note that aggressive handling may provoke VF, do not massage); at hospital, active rewarming w ICU monitor, hydration
- Frostnip: shelter from wind, warm affected area w/o rubbing, or immersion in warm water
- Frostbite: remove pt to warm facility; remove wet clothing; cover area w dry dressing until able to rx at medical facility w immersion in water at 40–42.2°C for 15–30 min. Cover blisters w aloe vera; give anlagesia, dt booster if appropriate
- Trench foot/chilblain: rapid rewarming in warm water

Prevent: Appropriate clothing/other protection (sleeping bag, bivy sack) etc. depending on availability of warm shelter; prefer close fit w/o constriction in clothes, w use of layers (polypropylene at skin surface; avoid cotton); keep well-hydrated, fed, avoid ETOH, and be aware of early sx of cold injury

---

7.5 ARTHROPOD BITES AND STINGS

Nejm 1994;331:523; J Am Acad Derm 1997;35:243

Cause: Contact w biting insects/arachnids, stinging insects (usually *Hymenoptera*), or skin contact w caterpillars, blister beetles, etc.

Epidem: Worldwide; *Hymenoptera* (bees/wasps) stings cause 40 deaths/yr in U.S.; rxns may occur to fire ants (Nejm 1990;323:462), scorpions, spiders; of note—*Latrodectus* species (black widow in U.S., other sp Africa, So Am, Eurasia); brown recluse spider in U.S., banana (So America); funnel web (Aust) spiders; violin spiders (brown recluse, etc.) recognize by violin shape on thorax; dangerous scorpions incl *Centruroides exilicaude* (Arizona, W Mexico), and 2 species in No Africa/Middle East/Sou Europe

Risk for travelers: Low, but incr w outdoor travel in tropics; domestic exposure a risk in some areas w scorpions/spiders

Pathophys: Allergic stings cause IgE-mediated rxn from weal and flare to anaphylaxis; rarely delayed serum sickness or other immune-mediated rxn (ie acute inflamm polyneuropathy; Jama 1982;247:1443); venomous insect bites rarely cause allergic rxn, but tissue rxn to particular toxins

Sx:

- Insect sting: acute localized pain, itch, red, swelling to generalized hives, wheezing, or dizziness
- Spider bite: pain, redness at bite, often delayed several hr; no itch; sometimes arthralgia, abdominal pain, or chest pain (widow spiders)
- Scorpion sting: immediate pain, swelling
- Mites (chiggers): tiny itchy papules at exposed sites
- Ticks: often no sx w bite; delayed local irritation, swelling, erythema in some

Si:

- Insect stings: redness, swelling, urticarial, systemic allergic si
- Spider bite: redness, swelling, often w central vesicle or local skin necrosis (brown spiders), regional muscle spasm (widow spiders), hypertension, autonomic nervous system si (salivation, lacrimation, vomiting) in funnel web spiders and banana spiders
- Scorpion sting: hyperesthesia w gentle tap at sting site; systemic rxn may evolve to include cranial nerve abnorm, somatic skeletal neuromuscular si
- Caterpillar contact dermatitis: linear erythema, vesicles, or urticaria

Complc: Insect stings can lead to life-threatening allergic rxn; spider bites to soft tissue necrosis, intravascular hemolysis, renal failure (Am J Clin Path 1995;104:463); fatal scorpion stings w *Centruroides exilicauda* (children <9 yo) in sw U.S., Mexico; tick bites rarely can cause tick paralysis (see 19.4)

Rx:

- Insect stings: cold compress, shake lotions (calamine w menthol); scrape off stinger; if systemic: for urticaria/pruritus only, and age >45, oral antihistamine; for additional systemic sx, give epinephrine sc (1:1000–0.1% or 1 mg/mL—0.3–0.5 mg); children (0.01 mL/kg); repeat in 15–20 min if w/o response

- Spider bites: cold compresses, analgesics; dapsone may have utility in severe loxoscelism (Jama 1983;250:648); antivenin locally available in some parts of world if spider idenified—can result in serum sickness rxn
- Scorpion stings: cold compresses or ice packs; hospitalize for systemic sx; for *Centruroides* stings, antevenom use controversial; serum sickness common w antivenom, but anaphylaxis rare (Ann Emerg Med 1999;34(5):615); IV midazolam infusion can be effective (Ann Emerg Med 1999;34(5):620)
- Caterpillar contact rxn: remove spines by application of adhesive tape; topical steroid
- Chiggers: rx itch w topical steroid, antihistamine
- Ticks: remove w forceps applied close to skin (Pediatrics 1985;75:997)

Prevent: Biting insects/arachnids (Ann IM 1998;128:931)

1. Bring protective clothing (ie, long sleeved shirts, pants, etc.) for use when biting insects are active; clothing may be treated (ie, wrists, ankles, etc.) w DEETcontaining repellants (see below) or permethrin
2. DEET (*N,N*-diethyl-3-methyl benzamide) containing repellants remain the most effective agents of over 20,000 compounds tested; safety is well-established w correct use; very rare reports of neurotoxicity (seizure, encephalopathy) in children given highly concentrated products over large surface areas); duration of activity on skin related to potency, but little additional benefit (and incr risk dermatitis) above 50% DEET; preparations w 20–35% DEET usually suffice
No evidence of clear assoc of toxicity w concentration (EPA); longer-acting repellants useful in tropics incl controlled release products, such as Ultrathon (12 hr efficacy), Sawyer Controlled Release, others; reapplication still required w swimming, heavy sweating
3. Application of permethrin insecticides to clothing (NOT skin) is a useful adjunct to DEET to decr contact w biting insects and ticks; permethin is safe, not harmful to fabrics, persists through washing
4. Bednets, esp when treated w permethrin, offer enhanced protection against night–biting mosquitos and reduce risk of malaria transmission (as well as discouraging bites by other insects, spiders, etc.; Lancet 1995;345:499); several types are available at camping/travel supply companies

5. Persons w hx serious allergic rxn should carry epinephrine syringe, have Medalert bracelet

7.6 VENOMOUS REPTILES

Guerrant et al, Trop Inf Dis, Churchill Livingstone, 1999, ch. 13; Ann Emerg Med 2001;37(2):166

Cause: Bites by any of 5 families of snakes that produce neurotoxins or hemotoxins

Epidem: Worldwide, except New Zealand, Hawaii, Madagascar, West Indies, other isolated island populations; cause 30,000–40,000 deaths/yr (WHO); most bites in children handling snakes or agricultural workers; in U.S., 95% rattlesnake bites occur on hands or feet (West J Med 1988;148:37); 20–50% of bites by venomous snakes may be "dry," w little or no venom; in U.S., 1000–2000 bites/yr w fatality <1%; in Costa Rica, est annual deaths due to snakebite is 3/100,000

Risk for travelers: Very rare, and usually overestimated; for tropical rainforest biologists working in Central/So America, estimate of 1 bite per 400,000 person-hrs in field (Natural History 1985;94:2); overall 2–20 × incr risk over U.S. of venomous snakebite in tropics

Sx: Variable, depend on toxin type; for pit vipers, immediate pain, soft tissue swelling; swelling may progress over 1–12 hr to involve entire limb; 6–24 hr hemorragic bullae; systemic sx incl nausea, vomiting, parethesias of scalp and face, faintness, petechiae, etc. cardiovascular sx (bradycardia, hypotension, hypertension), neuro sx follow; for elapids (ie, coral snakes, cobras, mambas, kraits, all Australian venom sp) often no inflammation/pain at site of bite; onset of neuro sx delayed (1–12 hr); then nausea weakness, muscle fasciculations, CN sx, paralysis, difficulty breathing; for burrowing asps: similar to pit vipers but less severe, except w coronary spasm (Toxicon 1986;24:285); for sea snake: similar to elapid, but w incr muscle pain

Si: As above; paired punctures may be visible on skin w venomous bite

Crs: variable, from localized tissue injury to cardiovascular collapse or flaccid paralysis; for pit vipers, coagulopathy w hypovolemias, intracranial hemorrhage (Am J Trop Med 1991;44:93)

Dx: Venom ELISA in use in some countries to identify species; killed snakes should be transported w care as bite reflex may persist for 1 hr

Rx: Victim should rest quietly until transport; field techniques for rx, incl suction, extractors, etc. of unproven efficacy (Nejm 1992;327:1322; Wilderness Env Med 2000;11:149); for elapid/sea snake bites, Australian compression/immobilization technique may be helpful (Med J Aust 1981;2:293; Ann Emerg Med 2001;37:168); consists of broad, moderately constrictive (40–70 mm Hg) bandage over most of affected limb w splint; anitvenins may be effective if species or genus of snake identified (Jama 1987;258:1615); most are equine serum based, w variable rates of hypersensitivity documented (Am J Trop Med 1998;58:22; Wilderness Env Med 2000;11:163); field use of currently available equine-based antivenom is discouraged

Prevent: Use of knee-high boots w field work; many tropical snakes are active at night, so use caution when walking after dark

7.7 MARINE ENVENOMATIONS

Am Fam Physician 1989;40:97; Guerrant et al, Trop Inf Dis, Churchill Livingstone 1999, ch. 13; Nejm 1991;325:486

Cause: Puncture wounds or stings (esp coelenterate nematocysts) from venom-containing sea life, incl jellyfish, anemones, coral, sea urchins, cone shells, fish, etc.

Epidem: Worldwide, esp in subtropic and tropical oceans and coastal areas; fatalities rare, but box jellyfish stings cause est 100 deaths/yr in IndoPacific region (J Trav Med 1998;5:135)

Risk for travelers: Minor dermatitic rxn (sea bather's eruption, etc.) not uncommon in vacationers to Caribbean resorts (Jama 1993;269:1669); sea urchin spine injuries, fire coral stings seen in snorkelers, scuba divers, esp w night dives; risk often inapparent, as larval organisms w nematocysts that carry stinging cells are not visible; fine tentacles of blue-bottle/Portuguese man-of-war up to 30 m long

Sx:
- Seabather's eruption: pruritic rash w/in 1 hr bathing under swimsuit (due to invisible jellyfish larvae w nematocysts, esp thimble jellyfish)

- Jellyfish stings: immediate stinging pain and redness in fine whip-like pattern; box jellyfish causes rapid cardiopulmonary arrest (Jama 1991;266:1404)
- Fire coral, anemone, bristleworm contact: similar, w/o long streaking pattern
- Sea urchin puncture: mild pain, irritation, and swelling/discoloration at puncture site
- Venomous fish (stingrays, scorpion, fish): immediate pain at site w swelling
- Blue-ring octopus bite: initial tingling/numbness becomes spreading pain w development of blurred vision, dysphagia, paralysis in 15–30 min
- Cone shell sting: localized sting; if severe, generalized neuro sx develop

Si:
- Seabather's eruption: follicular or urticarial/vesicular rash in distribution of swimsuit
- Jellyfish stings: linear vesicles or welts in characteristic pattern
- Sea urchin puncture: purple/black discoloration at puncture; can form granuloma
- Stingrays, etc.: tissue necrosis at wound site

Complc: Most are self-limited; sea urchin spine can cause synovitis if near joint; secondary infection can occur w all; life-threatening neurotoxic rxns subside in 24–48 hrs if pt can be supported

Rx:
- Seabather's eruption: clean area thoroughly, topical steroid
- Jellyfish, coral, anemome stings: immerse in 5% acetic acid, topical steroids (antivenin available for box jellyfish poisonings)
- Sponge/bristleworm irritations: immerse in 5% acetic acid; remove spicules w adhesive tape
- Sea urchin puncture: immerse in nonscalding hot water (45°C) for 30–90 min; spines that penetrate to joint or bone may need location w imaging; note thin spines in tissue are difficult to remove as they crumble w pressure
- Stingrays, fish punctures: immerse area in hot nonscalding water for 30–90 min; remove spine fragments; consider antivenin for severe stonefish envenomations
- Cone shell, blue-ringed octopus: ? pressure/immobilization technique (as in snakebite)

- *NOTE: Do Not Wash Stings w Fresh Water*; it triggers release of nematocyst toxin

Prevent: Wear water shoes when walking in shallow water tidal pools; if snorkeling, scuba, learn to recognize local marine dangers; do not handle live cone shells; showering w/o suit after swim prevents sea bather's eruption (Nejm 1993;329:542)

7.8 UNDERSEA DIVING-RELATED ILLNESS

Nejm 1992;326:30; J Travel Med 1999;6:180

Cause: Due to effect of changes in environmental pressure w descent/ascent; 1 atmosphere for for each 10 m; may cause barotrauma, decompression sickness

Epidem: 2 million certified divers in U.S.: approx 100 deaths/yr; 60% are drownings; 800 cases of decompression sickness (DCS) reported in 1994 in U.S.; divers with patent foramen ovale are 5× incr risk for presence of ischemic brain lesions on MRI, though lesions also seen in divers at higher than expected rate w/o patent foramen ovale (Ann IM 2001;134:21)

Risk for travelers: Incr risk DCS if air travel too soon after dives (see below); note that resort scuba courses may not adequately prepare; may ignore careful screening for underlying medical issues that make diving more hazardous

Pathophys: Barotrauma; pressure differences cause gas expansion/contraction in air-filled body cavities (ie, sinuses, middle/inner/ext ear, GI tract, lungs); rapid ascent w/o adequate exhalation lead to pulmonary overpressurization syndrome (POPS); other illness related to incr partial pressure nitrogen on deep dives and assoc nitrogen narcosis, and w too rapid ascent, DCS due to release of free nitrogen gas from supersaturation of tissues

Sx:
- Barotrauma (minor): otalgia, sinus pain; rare vertigo due to inner ear trauma
- POPS: dyspnea, pleurisy (if pneumothorax), dysphagia, crepitus
- Air embolism (severe cmplc of POPS): acute focal neuro changes on surfacing consistent with stroke

- Nitrogen narcosis: confusion, lack of concentration (at 70–90 ft or more)
- DCS type 1: onset 1–6 hr after surfacing; mottled pruritic rash, myalgias ("the bends")
- DCS type 2: blurred vision, CNS changes, paresthesias, weakness, paralysis, chest pain, vertigo, hearing loss ("the staggers")

Si:
- Barotrauma: hemorrhagic or perforated tympanic membrane
- POPS and arterial gas embolus (AGE): sc emphysema, focal neuro sx
- DCS: mottled (livedo) rash, esp on upper trunk; paraparesis, focal neuro si

Crs: DCS sx may persist mo, even with rx; focal neuro trauma may be permanent

Rx:
- Barotrauma: rest, O_2 (if nec), desist dives until complete recovery
- AGE: keep supine; O_2; evac for recompression
- DCS: keep supine; O_2; recompression

Prevent: Assure training/certification w rigorous scuba course; do not dive w medical contra-indications (active resp infx, other acute illness); all divers should have medical clearance, asthma, chronic pulmonary disease, seizure disorder, psychiatric illness all disqualify; divers need to use decompression tables precisely; no air travel w/in 12 hr of a shallow (nondecomp dive) or 24 hr if after multiple daily dives or deep dives; information available: Divers Alert Network: Emergency hotline (919-684-8111) or nonemerg (919-684-2948)

8 Illness During Transportation

8.1 MOTION SICKNESS/JET LAG

Lancet 1997;350:1611; Postgrad Med 1999;106:177

Cause: Motion sickness—conflicting inputs to CNS from visual/vestibular systems; jet lag—disruption of circadian rhythms by transmeridian flight travel

Epidem: Motion sickness—common; up to 60% children prone to car sickness; seasickness attack rates may reach 100% in rough weather; 1% average incidence w commercial air travel; sea travel highest risk; highest risk in children (age 3–12), women, passengers

Jet lag—Nearly universal w crossing of 3 or more time zones; increases w westbound travel relative to eastbound travel (human circadian rhythm is slightly >24 hr)

Risk for travelers: Motion sickness common w "rough" sea/air travel; jet lag common w transmeridian flights; increased risk jet lag w ETOH, lack of sleep, stress, number of time zones

Sx: Motion sickness—sighing, lassitude, salivation, eructation, nausea, dizziness, sweating; eventual vomiting

Jet lag—insomnia, fatigue, daytime drowsiness, apathy, irritability

Si: Motion sickness—pallor, sweating, pulse changes

Crs: MS—adaptation to provoking stimulus usual in 24–36 hr; persistent vomintg may dehydrate

Jl—adaptation to transmeridian flight takes 4–6 d; longer to reestablish circadian rhythm

Rx: MS—rest; watch horizon; if persistent vomiting, etc., promethazine (50 mg im or suppository)

Jl—adopt new time zone schedule; frequent short naps; avoid ETOH; takes 1 d/time zone

Prevent: MS—No proven efficacy to common traditional/folk remedies; chemoprophylaxis is often effective; scopolamine (Transderm scop patch; oral tab 0.4–0.8 mg) or any of several antihistamines (meclizine 25–50 mg 1 hr before departure; dimenhydrinate OTC; promethazine 25 mg bid for adults; buclizine)

Note that scopolamine may cause CNS sx (Jama 1982;247:3081) and vision blurring in elderly; antihistamines, esp promethazine, cause drowsiness; no apparent differences in efficacy for prevention among antihistamines (J Travel Med 1994;1:203)

Jet lag—nonpharmacologic use of light exposure particularly timed bright light exposure (Science 1989;244:1328); use in AM for eastward travel, PM for westward

Pharmacologic rx include melatonin 3–5 mg at 3 AM destination time 3 d prior, then qhs for 4 nights after arrival; may cause drowsiness, ha (Jama 1996:276:1011); benzodiazepines have been used to promote rest in flight, but episodes of transient amnesia reported in a few (Jama 1987;258:945)

8.2 DEEP VEIN THROMBOPHLEBITIS ("ECONOMY CLASS SYNDROME")

Lancet 1988;11:497; J Travel Med 2000;7:149; Br Med J 2001;322:188

Cause: Immobility (and perhaps leg compression by seat) leads to lower extremity venous thrombosis; hypobaric environment of air travel incr markers of activated coagulation 2×–8×

Epidem: Air travel may account for 5% of all DVT; risk ratio for travel was 4× incr in one study of acute DVT (Chest 1999;115:440) but w/o incr risk in another (Lancet 2000;356:1492); overall evidence of risk is circumstantial; risk is age >40, prior DVT, pregnancy, CHF, dehydration

Risk for travelers: Increased w duration of immobility, length of drive/flight w/o stop; mean time associated w DVT was 5 hr (Chest 1999;115:440)

Sx: Leg pain (esp calf); swelling of ankle, calf, or thigh; dyspnea; pleurisy; syncope if PE

Si: Greater than 1 cm difference in lower leg diameter at calf; tenderness of calf, thigh (esp adductor canal)

Crs: W/o immediate rx, progressive clot formation, risk of PE

Rx: Anticoagulation w heparin, enoxaparin followed by Coumadin for 3–6 mo; leg elevation

Prevent: Interrupt sitting on long car/train/plane trips w ambulation q 2 hr; leg stretching exercises; prophylaxis w/ aspirin or other agents has been recommended by some for high risk travelers, but no data of efficacy available

9 Protection of Special Groups

9.1 THE PREGNANT TRAVELER

Inf Dis Clin N Am 1998;12:325

KEY FACTORS

- Safety of travel
- Safety of immunizations
- Malaria prevention
- Prevention/management of traveler's diarrhea

SAFETY OF TRAVEL

Routine travel considered safe w exc of complicated pregnancy (see Table 9.1); fetal oxygen desaturation not observed w commercial air travel (Aviation Space Environmental Medicine 1976;47:77); however, airlines discourage travel at >35 wks (require letter); some conditions (ie, sickle cell anemia) problematic w decreased O_2 sats w air travel; DVT is a concern in pregnancy w/ air/car travel; recommend max duration 6 hr w car stops q 2 hr, at least, for ambulation; maternal trauma w car travel is greatest risk to fetus; use 3-point seat belt restraint w belt over low pelvis.

Table 9.1. Relative contraindications to international travel during pregnancy

Patients with obstetrical risk factors
- History of miscarriage
- Incompetent cervix
- History of ectopic pregnancy (ectopic with present pregnancy should be ruled out prior to travel)
- History of premature labor or premature rupture of membranes
- History of or present placental abnormalities
- Threatened abortion or vaginal bleeding during present pregnancy
- Multiple gestation in present pregnancy
- History of toxemia, hypertension, or diabetes with any pregnancy
- History of infertility or difficulty becoming pregnant
- Primigravida >35 years of age or <15 years of age

Patients with general medical risk factors
- Valvular heart disease or congestive heart failure
- History of thromboembolic disease
- Severe anemia
- Chronic organ system dysfunction requiring frequent medical interventions

Patients contemplating travel to destinations that may be hazardous
- High altitudes
- Areas endemic for or with ongoing outbreaks of life-threatening food- or insect-borne infections
- Areas where chloroquine-resistant *Plasmodium falciparum* is endemic
- Areas where live-virus vaccines are required and recommended

Adapted from Health Information for International Travel, Centers for Disease Control.

SAFETY OF IMMUNIZATIONS

Preferable to vaccinate before pregnancy, or after first trimester; however, risk of some travel-related diseases is inc in pregnancy (ie hepatitis A, influcnza). Decision based on individual risk/benefit (see Table 9.2); avoid live vaccines if possible. (Note in yellow fever outbreak w high risk, yellow fever vaccine given to 100 pregnant women w/o adverse effects (Trans Roy Soc Trop Med Hyg 1993;87:337).

Table 9.2. Vaccination during pregnancy

Type	Vaccine	Use during pregnancy
Cholera	Inactivated bacterial	Data on safety in pregnancy are not available*
Hepatitis A	Inactivated virus	Data on safety in pregnancy are not available
Hepatitis B	Subunit virus	Administer if indicated
Immune globulins, pooled or hyperimmune	Immune globulin or specific globulin preparations	Administer if indicated
Influenza	Inactivated whole virus or subunit	Administer if indicated
Japanese encephalitis	Inactivated virus	Data on safety in pregnancy are not available*
Measles	Live-attenuated virus	Contraindicated
Meningococcal meningitis	Polysaccharide	Administer if indicated
Mumps	Live-attenuated virus	Contraindicated
Plague	Inactivated bacterial	Data on safety in pregnancy are not available*
Polio, inactivated	Inactivated virus	Administer if indicated
Polio, oral	Live-attenuated virus	Administer if indicated
Rabies	Inactivated virus	Administer if indicated
Rubella	Live-attenuated virus	Administer if indicated
Tetanus-diphtheria	Toxoid	Administer if indicated
Typhoid	Inactivated bacterial	Data on safety in pregnancy are not available
Varicella	Live-attenuated virus	Contraindicated
Yellow fever	Live-attenuated virus	Administer if indicated

* Should weigh the theoretical risk of vaccination against the risk of disease.
Adapted from Health Information for International Travel, Centers for Disease Control.

MALARIA PREVENTION

Malaria during pregnancy causes increased fetal loss (Am J Trop Med Hyg 1996;55:61); susceptibility to clinical malaria incr during pregnancy and 2 mo postpartum (Nejm 2000;343:598). Pregnant women should carefully consider risk/benefit of elective travel in malarious areas; if traveling (or residing) in malarious area, observe strict practices re: prevention of mosquito bites as outlined in section 7.5 (ie, minimize outdoor evening exposure, use screens/bed nets; DEET-containing repellants, if used sparingly on exposed skin in low to moderate concentrations are generally considered safe); note that pregnant women attract 2× mosquitos than nonpregnant (Lancet 2000;355:1972); chloroquine is considered safe in pregnancy (BMJ 1985;290:1466); can use in the few areas w choroquine-sensitive malaria or combine w proguanil (not available as single agent in U.S.) for resistant areas, but this combination less effective than mefloquine (Lancet 1993;341:1299); mefloquine appears safe when used in 2nd to 3rd trimesters (JID 1994;169:595); although teratogenicity not observed w inadvertent mefloquine use in 1st trimester (JID 1997;176:831), it should be avoided during 1st trimester and 3 mo before pregnancy. Primaquine and doxycycline use are contraindicated. Malarone is currently not approved for use in pregnancy.

PREVENTION/RX TRAVELER'S DIARRHEA

Dehydration due to enteric infx is risky in pregnancy; it is advisable to carry oral rehydration solution (ORS—see Table 9.3) and to use caution in food and restaurant selection; water should be boiled; short-term iodine use is acccptable; loperamide or diphenoxylate (category B drugs) can be given, w antibiotics for rx of diarrhea. Bismuth subsalicylate should be avoided. Safe antibiotics for use in pregnancy for traveler's diarrhea incl trimethoprim/sulfa (but can cause kernicterus in late pregnancy) and the macrolides erythromycin (exc the estolate) and azithromycin (category B); oral amoxicillin or cephalosporin safe but efficacy not established.

Table 9.3. Composition of World Health Organization oral rehydration solution (ORS) for diarrheal illness

Ingredient	Amount (g/L)
Sodium chloride	3.5
Potassium chloride	1.5
Glucose	20.0
Trisodium citrate*	2.9

* An earlier formulation that used sodium bicarbonate 2.5 g/L had a shorter shelf life, but was physiologically equivalent and may still be produced in some countries.
Adapted from Health Information for International Travel, Centers for Disease Control.

9.2 THE HIV POSITIVE TRAVELER

Ann Intern Med 1991;114:582; CID 2000;31:1403; Inf Dis Clin NA 1998;12:369

KEY FACTORS

- Incr susceptibility to (some) infx
- Vaccination efficacy/safety
- Drug interactions
- Government restrictions

SUSCEPTIBILITY TO INFX

Major concern is incr susceptibility to prolonged/relapsing and bacteremic infx due to bacterial enteric pathogens (esp salmonella, campylobacter—Ann Intern Med 1988;108:540); risk of salmonella inc 100× over controls in NYC (CID 1994;18:358); enteric parasites also a concern if CD4 count low, esp cryptosporidia, isospora, cyclospora. Also at incr risk from pneumococcus, M. tb; and of chronic disseminated infx from fungi (histoplasmosis, blastomycosis, coccidioidomycosis, paracoccidioidomycosis, penicilliosis) and some parasites (ie, Chagas, visceral leishmaniasis). For prevention of enteric infx, use treated water (and consider additional filtration) in developing countries w standard #53 (absolute filter) to remove parasitic cysts not killed by chlorine. Use of quinolone for prophylaxis may be considered for short-term travel, and all should carry rx dose of quinolone or other effective antibiotic (ie, azithromycin, etc.).

VACCINE EFFICACY/SAFETY

May have inadequate immune response to vaccination, esp w low CD4 (Nejm 1987;316:683); but all routine vaccinations updated unless contraindicated (as w some live vaccines); should have current pneummovax, Td, influenza; hep A and B if not already immune; strongly consider typhoid (not live) if going to developing countries; killed polio vaccine (IEPV) if indicated; live vaccines are problematic; can give MMR if CD4 >200 and at risk (note 1 case measles pneumonitis from MMR in HIV pt w low CD4; MMWR 1993;45:603); yellow fever vaccine contraindicated, but has been given to small # (<100) pts w CD4 >200 w/o adverse effect (J Travel Med 1995;2:145); avoid BCG.

DRUG INTERACTIONS

Esp significant w use of protease inhibitor containing regimens; effect w mefloquine unkown, but difficulties may occur w ritonavir (doxycycline or malarone should be good alternatives for malaria prophylaxis); attention should also be paid to timing of antirctroviral rx (w or w/o meals, etc.) and adequate supplies in 2 different bags as it may be difficult to replace medications overseas. Use of UVA & UVB sunscreen is recommended given incr likelihood of photosensitivity rxns w use of multiple medications.

GOVERNMENT RESTRICTIONS

Pts should check entry requirements for participating nations, esp
   if planning long stay (nearly 50 countries restrict entry); see
   http://travel.state.gov./HIVtestingreqs.html; for additional information
   see: http://www.cdc.gov/travel/hivtrav.htm

9.3 THE PEDIATRIC TRAVELER

KEY FACTORS:

- Travel with very young children
- Immunizations
- Malaria
- Traveler's diarrhea

TRAVEL WITH VERY YOUNG CHILDREN

Travel with very young children to some areas of the world may be
   problematic. There are certain vaccines that cannot be given to young
   infants because of safety concerns or lack of efficacy. Young infants
   will have just started receiving the routinely recommended vaccines.
   They will not be adequately protected against many infections that
   may be common in the areas of travel. Prophylaxis against malaria, a
   disease that may be particularly severe in the very young, is difficult.
   Young children are at increased risk for serious bacterial infections
   and immediate medical evaluation is recommended for young infants
   with signs such as fever, lethargy, and poor feeding. Diarrheal illness
   may rapidly lead to dehydration. Appropriate medical facilities may
   not be easily accessible for the traveler.

SPECIAL GROUPS

IMMUNIZATIONS (see also Chapter 3)

During the preparation for travel, the child's immunization record should be reviewed and updated as necessary. Vaccines that are not routinely recommended in childhood but may be indicated for travel are discussed below.

Hepatitis A: There are 2 hepatitis A vaccines that are currently available in the U.S. They both have pediatric and adult formulations.

Vaccine	Dose	Age	Vol.	Schedule
Havrix	720 ELU	2–18 y	0.5 mL	initial, 6–12 mo later
Vaqta	25 U	2–17 y	0.5 mL	initial, 6–18 mo later

Vaccination is considered protective 2–4 weeks after administration. Intramuscular immune globulin (IG) may be given to travelers with imminent departures. The recommended doses are listed below.

For children <2 years of age intramuscular immune globulin (IG) is recommended for protection against hepatitis A. The dose is 0.02 mL/kg for travel less than 3 months and 0.06 mL/kg for travel of 3–5 months duration. For extended periods of travel, 0.06 mg/kg is given every 5 months.

Typhoid: Risk is greater in children than adults. There are currently two typhoid vaccines available in the U.S. The Vi capsular polysaccharide vaccine may be used for children ≥2 years of age. It is given intramuscularly. The other vaccine is the live-attenuated Ty21a vaccine. One capsule is given orally every 2 days for a total of 4 capsules. It may be prescribed for children who are ≥6 years of age and not immunocompromised. It should not be given within 24 hours of an antimicrobial agent.

Because currently there is not available immunization for children <2 years of age, parents should be cautioned about food and water precautions. Breastfeeding may offer some additional protection in young children. Note that the recently developed conjugate vaccine may be the most effective option for children when it becomes available (Nejm 2001;344:1263)

Yellow fever: Because of a potential risk of vaccine-associated encephalitis, there are specific cautions about administration of yellow fever vaccine in young children. The vaccine is recommended for children ≥9 months of age who are traveling to areas where yellow fever immunization is required or suggested. Children who are 6–9 months of age should only be vaccinated if they will be in areas of epidemic yellow fever and a high level of protection against mosquito bites cannot be achieved. In exceptional circumstances, children 4–6 months of age may be immunized after consultation with the CDC. Children <4 months of age may not receive this vaccine. It is also contraindicated in children with hypersensitivity to eggs or immunosuppression.

Japanese encephalitis: The Japanese encephalitis vaccine may be given to children ≥1 year of age. For children <3 years of age, the vaccine dose is 0.5 mL given subcutaneously on days 0, 7, and 30. The usual dose of 1 mL is given to children ≥3 years of age. The vaccine series should be completed at least 10 days before departure because of the possibility of delayed reactions.

Meningococcal: The quadrivalent vaccine available in the U.S. may be given to children >2 years of age who are traveling to areas with epidemic meningococcal disease.

Rabies: Risk incr in children over adults. Children may receive prophylaxis against rabies. Parents should be advised to keep children away from stray animals and to seek immediate medical care if significant contact occurs.

MALARIA (see also Chapter 4)

Prophylaxis against malaria is more difficult in children. Some medications are not recommended for use in children whereas other medications do not have pediatric formulations. It is recommended that for accurate dosing in young children of medications such as mefloquine and choroquine that the prescriptions are filled at a compounding pharmacy. Capsules containing the precise dose can be prepared. The capsules can then be opened and the drug mixed with something sweet such as chocolate syrup or applesauce. These drugs should be in childproof containers away from children. Parents should be advised of the dangers of overdose.

It is recommended that insect repellant containing ≤10% DEET be used for young children.

TRAVELER'S DIARRHEA (see also Chapter 5)

The use of antibiotics to prevent traveler's diarrhea is not generally recommended. Adequate hydration should be maintained in children with diarrhea. Oral rehydration solutions may be used. Children who develop high fevers, bloody diarrhea, or dehydration should be brought to a medical facility. Some authorities recommend treatment of mild to moderate traveler's diarrhea in children w azithromycin (10 mg/kg on day 1, 5 mg/kg on days 2, 3), trimethroprim-sulfa (though widespread resistance to this drug limits effectiveness) or a single-dose of quinolone, though not FDA-approved for pediatric use (CID 2000;31:1079). Antimotility agents should not be prescribed for children <2 yr. In children >2 yr loperamide may be considered.

HIGH ALTITUDE TRAVEL

For information on travel with young children to high altitudes, see Arch. Pediatr Adolesc Med 1998;152:683

9.4 THE DIABETIC TRAVELER

Postgrad Med 1999;105:111; Inf Dis Clin N Am 1998;12:386

KEY FACTORS

- Circadian/schedule disruption
- Documentation and supplies
- Environmental stressors
- Skin/other infx

CIRCADIAN/SCHEDULE DISRUPTIONS

Flexibility required w changes in time, meals, etc. IDDM pts may benefit from use of insulin lispro (Humalog) for quick use just before meals in place of regular insulin given more rapid effect; new delivery systems that are compact (ie, insulin pens) are helpful, as may be availability of glucagon pens for hypoglycemic rxn; no data that meridian-related insulin adjustments are necessary.

DOCUMENTATION/SUPPLIES

Letters from physician w information on diabetic schedules and reserve prescription are suggested. Take double expected needed supplies w carry-on luggage. Have carbohydrates available during flights (along w insulin, glucagon, testing equipment, etc.). Use Med Alert bracelet. ADA (below) produces *Buyer's Guide to Diabetic Supplies* w info on international availability of supplies.

ENVIRONMENTAL STRESSORS

Metabolic dysregulation common w travel to tropics (J Travel Med 1999;6:12); diabetics should be prepared for dose adjustments. Cold climates also may require change; accuracy of testing meters may be less at high altitude (Diabetes Education 1989;15:144)

SKIN/OTHER INFX

Staph skin infx may be more freq in tropical climates; pyomyositis, a rare condition in the U.S., is common in tropical areas; traveler's diarrhea poses additional challenges to diabetics—a plan should be in place for hydration rx

Additional information: American Diabetes Assoc (800-806-7801) http//www:diabetes.org

SPECIAL GROUPS

Section III

RECOGNITION AND TREATMENT OF TRAVEL-RELATED ILLNESS

10 The Traveler with Fever

Guerrant Trop Inf Dis 1999;Ch 125:1381; Inf Dis Clin N Am
    1998;12:445

OVERVIEW

Self-limited fever common (2%) in short-term travelers from
    industrialized countries to developing countries (JID 1987;156:84).
    Challenge for clinicians in returning traveler w fever is to determine
    significance and diagnostic approach efficiently. Diseases may be
    unrelated to particular geographies of travel in $^1/_2$ (Q J Med
    1995;88:277), but may include potentially life-threatening tropical
    infections in a substantial number. Malaria accounts for 30–60% of
    fevers in returning tropical travelers in several hospital- or clinic-
    based series (Q J Med 1995;88:277; Trav Med Adv 1994;5:27;
    BMJ 1978;1:966); 20–30% remained undiagnosed; 1–5% of cases
    attributed to other tropical diseases (esp dengue, typhoid, enteric
    infections, viral hepatitis, rickettsial disease). Risk of tropical infx incr
    w duration of travel, outdoor activities, adventurous itinerary. Types
    of infx considerations differ w geography of travel (see Appendix 1).
    Several excellent reviews of considerations by geography include
    Africa (Nejm 1993;328:1061), SE Asia/Oceania (Curr Clin Top Inf
    Dis 1992;12:138), SW Asia/Middle East (Curr Clin Top Inf Dis
    1993;13:57), Latin America (Curr Clin Top Inf Dis 1993;13:26).
    See also Wilson, *Guide to World Infections*, Oxford University Press,
    1991

TRAVELER WITH FEVER

Critical data to consider:
- Geographic exposure (countries and areas visited; rural vs urban)
- Time since exposure (incubation period)
- Behavioral exposure (type of activities, exp to arthropods, sexual contact, etc.)
- Use of medications (antimalarials, antibiotics, other)
- Immunization hx
- Duration of travel, prior travel/residential hx (ie, immune vs nonimmune)
- Co-existence of other sx and si (ie, careful hx/PE for rash, etc.)

Major considerations by possible incubation period:
- W/in 2 wks of exposure: MALARIA (18.25); dengue and other arboviruses (20.1, 20.2, 20.5); rickettsial infections (16.39, 16.52); typhoid and other enteric fevers (16.51); rarely, viral hemorrhagic fevers (Lassa, etc.), anthrax, plague, tularemia, psittacosis, leptospirosis, meningococcal disease, relapsing fever, yellow fever, alphaviruses, etc.
- W/in 1 month of exposure, but >2 wks: MALARIA; typhoid, viral hepatitis (A, C, E), rickettsial disease, leptospirosis, amebic liver abcess, various enteric infx; rarely brucellosis, HIV, rabies, schistosomiasis, tuberculosis, etc.
- Greater than 1 month postexposure: MALARIA; viral hepatitis (A, B, C, E); rarely schistosomiasis (Katayama fever syndrome, others; see 18.26), filariasis (18.17), brucellosis, tbc, fungal infections, leishmaniasis, amebic liver abcess, parasitic flukes, HIV, melioidosis, etc.

Major considerations with fever and rash: Dengue (20.5), rickettsial diseases (16.39, 16.52), meningococcus (16.27), leptospirosis (16.22), various viral diseases (ie, alphaviruses [see 20.1], HIV, if unimmunized: measles, rubella, varicella); w hemorrhagic rashes soon after return from an endemic area, consider viral hemorrhagic fevers (20.3, 20.4, 20.6, 20.13); allergic drug rashes are not uncommon; w urticarial rashes consider also viral hepatitis, schistosomiasis

Major considerations with fever and diarrhea: MALARIA; enteric bacterial infx (esp salmonellosis, campylobacter), *C. difficile* colitis, amebic dysentery, other enteric protozoans (ie, cyclospora, isospora, etc.). (See 18.2, 18.11, 18.12)

Major considerations with fever and mental status change: MALARIA; meningococcal or other bacterial meningitis (16.27), rickettsial diseases (16.39, 16.52), arboviral encephalitis (20.2), spirochetal disease (incl syphilis, relapsing fever, Lyme, leptospirosis), African trypanosomiasis (18.1), chronic meningitis due to tuberculosis, fungal, brucella infx; if eosinophilic meningitis, consider *Angiostrongylus cantonensis* (18.5)

Initial diagnostic approach in returning travelers with fever:

- If malaria exposure by hx, look for malaria w thick/thin blood smear or rapid antigen test (see 18.25); if initial smear is negative, repeat × 3 over 6–12 hr; if parasites present, assume *P. falciparum* malaria unless reliably shown to be otherwise; admit for hydration, initiation of rx, and monitor until drop in parasitemia confirmed
- In addition to careful hx/PE, check CBC w diff, liver enzymes, blood cultures on all
- If patient has petechial/purpuric rash, and viral hemorrhagic fever a consideration on basis of incubation period, itinerary, etc, consider isolation until dx made
- When the dx is not apparent, review Ddx in light of travel hx and as if there was no travel hx; repeat hx/PE regularly
- In severely ill pts, w appropriate travel hx, empiric rx for malaria, rickettsial disease, in addition to usual broad-spectrum antibiotic coverage should be considered until negative data can be assured, particularly when lab is inexperienced; seek advice from ID consultant if possible.

11 The Traveler with Diarrhea

Inf Dis Clin N Am 1998;12:489

OVERVIEW

30–40% of U.S. travelers to tropical countries develop diarrheal illness; most are self-limited, often due to enterotoxigenic *E. coli*, last 4–5 d or less w rx. Diarrhea persisting >2 wk is unusual; usually reflects the presence of more persistent bacterial pathogens (ie, campylobacter, salmonella, etc.), parasitic protozoa (ie, giardia, ameba, cyclospora, etc.) or development of *C. difficile* due prior anitibiotic treatment; however, temporary lactose intolerance developing after enteric infections is commonly overlooked. Of 10,000 Latin American travelers, only 3% had diarrhea lasting >2 wk, 1–2% longer than one mo (CID 1996;22:124)

Criticial data to consider:
- Geography of possible exposure (frequency of particular enteric pathogens high in some regions (ie, giardia in Russia; vibrios in Japan, Thailand; cyclospora in Nepal)
- Assoc sx (ie, presence of fever raises likelihood of invasive enteric bacteria or ameba; *C. difficile*; weight loss incr likelihood of giardia, cryptosporidia, etc.)
- Remember malaria/other systemic illnesses may have prominent GI sx
- Details of possible food/water exposures (esp raw seafood or meats)
- Type of diarrhea (ie, "dysenteric" w cramps/tenesmus/bloody diarrhea vs watery, voluminous diarrhea)
- Preexisting risk factors for nontravel-related GI disease

Major considerations with watery diarrhea >2 wk (w/o fever): Persistent enteric bacteria (esp salmonella, campylobacter; see 16.9, 16.16, 16.28, 16.30, 16.51, 16.53), protozoal infx (esp giardia, ameba, cryptosporidia, microsporidia, cyclospora; see 18.2, 18.11, 18.12, 18.20), C. difficile, lactose intolerance (16.34), "postinfectious bacterial overgrowth"; note that flouroquinolone-resistant campylobacter is incr recognized cause of relapsing diarrhea in travelers to SE Asia.

Major considerations w diarrhea assoc w fever: Always consider malaria, other systemic or generic intraabdominal process; invasive enteric bacteria (ie, salmonella, campylobacter); C. difficile, some enteric protozoa (ie, ameba, possibly cyclospora); rarely typhoid fever; consider less common enteric bacteria in particular regions (ie, aeromonas in travelers from Thailand (JID 1981;143:767), vibrios in Asian travelers (16.51), yersinia in travelers to Northern Europe (16.53); rarely helminths are a consideration (ie, schistosomiasis, trichinosis)

Major considerations in the patient w bloody diarrhea: Campylobacter, shigella, enterohemorrhagic, enteroinvasive E. coli, salmonella, aeromonas, yersinia, ameba, *Balantidium coli* (18.2), C. difficile (16.34)

Initial approach to management of persistent diarrhea:
- For pts w/o systemic sx: stool culture ×2; fresh stool specimen ×2 for parasitology (incl AFB stains for cyclospora, cryptosporidia, isospora; O + P or antigen detection assays for giardia, ameba); stool for C. difficile toxin, CBC (eosinophilia w isospora, strongyloides, schistosomiasis, etc.), LFTs (ameba, liver flukes); restrict lactose; if above negative, consider empiric trial of metronidazole (for ameba/giardia/c diff/overgrowth synd); sx persisting >30 d w/o dx merit cont'd GI workup w endoscopy (small bowel bx); in some travelers (ie, Nepal trekkers, others), an empiric course of Tm/S may be worthwhile to cover for undx cyclospora (and rare isospora)
- For initial management of pts w diarrhea/fever: blood smears for malaria if at risk, blood cultures ×2–3, stool cx ×2, stool for C. difficile toxin, stool for parasitologic exam (r/o ameba, cyclospora); CBC (high leukocytosis w invasive bacteriologic disease; eosinophilia w schisto, etc.); consider amebic serology; if no dx, and colitic sx, flexible sig w bx of any abnormal tissue

- For initial management of pts w bloody diarrhea: stool cultures ×2, stool for *C. difficile* toxin, *E. coli* 0157 toxin; stool for parasitology as above; blood cultures; amebic serology, CBC, LFTs; consideration of flexible sigmoidoscopy depending on course
- Rarely, chronic diarrhea may persist despite negative w/u; considerations include idiopathic "Brainerd diarrhea" (characterized by secretory diarrhea w focal, chronic inflammation on bowel bx) and tropical sprue (or tropical enteropathy) w villous flattening on small bowel bx (see 21.4); the former resolves spontaneously over 1 yr, the latter responds to 6 mo rx w tetracycline and folate (Ann Intern Med 1966;65:1201)

12 The Traveler with Skin Lesions

Inf Dis Clin N Am 1998;12:471

OVERVIEW

Skin rashes are commonly reported in retrospective surveys of travelers, though most are self-limited minor ailments (ie, sunburn and other phototoxic/sensitive reactions, insect bites, intertrigo, or prickly heat). Lesions that result in medical evaluation on return noted in one series (CID 1995;20:542) incl cutaneous larva migrans (25%), pyodermas incl staph/strep ecthyma (18%), arthropod reactive dermatoses (10%), myiasis (9%), tungiasis (6%), urticaria (5%), febrile syndromes w rash (4%), cutaneous leishmaniasis (3%). Likelihood of exotic causes for rashes varies w geography, type of trip, risk behavior, duration of travel, etc. Cutaneous larva migrans, common in beach sitters, may be rare in the rainforest ecotourist who returns w myiasis. A careful hx/PE may provide the clue to a phototoxic rxn to limes, a tick-borne rickettsial eschar in a safari survivor, or the swimsuit rash of "sea bather's eruption."

Critical data to consider:
- Onset of rash (circumstances of its appearance, duration, evolution)
- Activities of traveler (outdoor vs indoor, type of recreation, etc.)
- Itinerary of places visited (incl rural vs urban, beaches, unusual habitats)
- Anatomic location of rash (sun exposed or not; feet only, etc.)
- Pattern of rash (linear, clusters, single nodule, etc.)
- Morphology of lesions (papules, vesicles, ulcers, petechiae etc.)

- Presence of assoc sx (esp fever; see Chapter 10)
- Use of medications, sunscreens, insect repellants etc.

Major considerations w fever and rash, esp if petechial/hemorrhagic:
Dengue (20.5), other arbo- or alphavirus infx (20.1, 20.2), rickettsial infections (RMSF, tick typhus, scrub typhus; see 16.39, 16.41), meningococcemia and other bacterial sepsis (16.27), leptospirosis (16.22), rat-bite fever (16.37), viral hemorrhagic fevers (20.3, 20.4, 20.6, 20.13); note that any systemic infx w thrombocytopenia (ie, malaria) may have this appearance; as in U.S., enteroviral infx (echo, coxsackievirus); note that erythema multiforme rashes can have variable appearance and may be triggered by common infections (HSV, EBV, hep B, Grp A strep) along w drug allergy

Major considerations w papular eruptions: Insect bites (usually on exposed areas or borders w clothing; persistent lesions common w chiggers); papular urticaria may complicate insect bites w recurrent pruritic lesions; scabies (esp w substandard lodging, young travelers; see 19.3); allergic drug eruptions; for swimmers, consider cercarial dermatitis (see 18.26), sea bather's eruption (7.7); miliaria (spares hair follicles, on covered areas), folliculitis (esp "hot tub" *Pseudomonas* version on return from ski resorts, etc.); persistent pruritic eruption in long-term travelers/immigrants from endemic areas should prompt consideration of onchocerciasis (W Africa, C & So America; see 18.19), bartonellosis (Andes Mountains; see 16.5), leprosy (16.21), venereal syphilis/yaws, etc. (16.44)

Major considerations w persistent nodules (solitary or multiple):
Furunculosis (staph, etc.), myaisis (often movement w/in lesion is noted; see 19.2), tungiasis (Africa, C & So America; see 19.5); in genital areas, chancroid (16.11), LGV (16.25), syphilis (16.44); various systemic parasitoses, usually in assoc w eosinophilia; systemic fungal infection, mycobacteria (16.2), etc.; in divers, consider sea urchin spine (7.7), etc.

Major considerations w migratory swellings/skin lesions: Cutaneous larva migrans (slow, serpiginous; see 18.23), strongyloidiasis (fast, often on buttocks; eosinophilia; see 18.27); urticaria from any cause (lesions change q 24 hr); rarely *Loa loa* (Africa; see 18.18), gnathostomiasis (Thailand, Japan, Mexico; see 18.21), fascioliasis, paragonimiasis (18.10), sparganosis

Major considerations w ulcerative skin lesions: Pyodermas (ecthyma due to staph/strep), spider bites (brown recluse, others), secondary infection of insect bites; in genital areas, consider chancroid (16.11), syphilis (16.44), LGV (16.25); in biologists, ecotourists/adventure travelers, consider leishmaniasis (painless w rolled up edges; see 18.24); also consider eschar of rickettsial infx at tick bite if acutely ill or febrile (16.39, 16.52); rare causes in immigrants/expatriates may incl phagedenic tropical ulcer (anerobic infx, foul smelling), *Buruli* ulcer (mycobacterial; see 16.2), cutaneous diphtheria (16.15), anthrax (16.1), yaws (16.44), etc.; rarely seen on arrival in nonendemic countries are the chagoma of Chagas (18.9), chancre of African trypanosomiasis (18.1), cutaneous ambebiasis

Initial approach to management:
- For febrile pt, immediate evaluation usually prudent (see prior section)
- For others, careful hx/PE often gives answer; reassure pt that most skin eruptions in short-term travelers are self-limited and can rx symptomatically
- Genital lesions require thorough exam to r/o STDs
- Tropical travelers w undx skin lesion should have initial CBC (r/o eosinophilia), other lab as determined by Ddx
- Chronic ulcerative lesions usually require bx to r/o serious causes
- All patients w travel-acquired skin lesions need continued f/u until resolution

Note also the entity of delusional parasitosis in persons w/ or w/o travel history (see 21.2)

13 The Traveler with Eosinophilia

Inf Dis Clin N Am 1998;503

OVERVIEW

Eosinophilia (defined as >450 eosinophils per microliter in peripheral
   blood) in the returning traveler suggests the possibility of helminthic
   infection. The most common cause of eosinophilia world-wide is
   helminthic infections and the most common cause in industrial
   nations is atopic (allergic) disease. The absence of eosinophilia does
   not rule out parasitic infection. Protozoal infections are not generally
   associated with eosinophilia. Other causes include drug reactions,
   especially to antimalarials or antibiotics, and allergic disorders.
   Eosinophils increase in number with tissue invasion by helminths.
   Those infections with migrating larva have especially high eosinophil
   counts. High levels are seen in trichinosis, visceral larva migrans,
   ascaris when it is migrating, strongyloidiasis, filariasis, as well as
   schistosomiasis.

Helminths that are intralumenal in the bowel without tissue migration
   generally do not cause eosinophilia. After treatment of helminthic
   infections, eosinophilia may remain for several months. Eosinophils
   normally account for only 1–3% of peripheral blood leukocytes.
   The normal range is usually 350 cells per cubic millimeter of blood.
   Parasitic infections that cause eosinophilia are usually limited to
   helminthic parasites with the exception of two enterprotozoals:
   Isospora belli and *Dientamoeba fragilis*.

Critical data to consider:
- Geographic exposure (countries visited, endemic areas for particular helminths)
- Environmental exposure (swimming in fresh water, insect exposure, animal contact)
- Medication history while traveling
- Diarrheal illness while traveling
- Other symptomatic illness (rashes, wheezing, fevers, etc.)
- Duration of travel

Diagnostic studies: An initial evaluation in all patients, whether asx or not, usually includes confirmation of eosinophilia w a manual blood count to obtain an absolute eosinophil count; any drug that can be safely discontinued should be; a urinalysis w microscopic exam, LFTs, chest x-ray, PPD and stool for O + P exam ×3 are usually obtained

Quantitative serum immunoglobulins may also be ordered, along w a fresh stool to be examined for strongyloides larvae; other studies may be in ordered depending on the results of these initial studies and exposure hx; results of diagnostic studies may differ in nonimmune (short-term travelers, etc.) vs chronically exposed residents of a tropical country; w lower parasite loads, nonimmunes may have high eosinophilia w/o easily demonstrable parasites; if there are no focal findings to direct the w/u, and initial studies are unrevealing, serologic tests for schistosomiasis, strongyloidiasis, filariasis, etc. may be helpful (see 18.10, 18.16, 18.17, 18.26, 18.27, 18.30)

Specific parasitologic testing:
- Intestinal helminths and protozoals—do 3 stool examinations, one every other d; remember, many helminthic infections have a prepatent period before the appearance of eggs or larva in the stool; upper small bowel pathogens such as liver flukes (18.6), hookworms, strongyloides (18.29) may require small bowel bx or endoscopy, rectal biopsy for *Schistosoma haematobium* (18.26); filariasis diagnosis by concentrated blood specimens and filter examinations (pay attention to diurnal parasite cycle). (See 18.17)
- For skin lesions, skin snips or bx may prove helpful (18.19), though angioedematous lesions (ie, Calabar swellings, etc.) should not be biopsied

EOSINOPHILIA

- When indicated by respiratory sx, examine sputum for *paragonimiasis*, or occasionally, larvae of ascaris, or strongyloides; urine for schistosomiasis
- Charcot–Leyden crystals are often nondiagnostic but sometimes seen in helminthic infections. CSF positive for eosinophils in certain helminthic infections with CSF eosinophils consider cerebral cysticercosis (18.13), echinococcosis (18.14), angiostrongylus (18.3), gnathostomiasis (18.21). Nonparasitic causes of eosinophils include: TB, syphilis, drug reactions, and coccidioidomycosis (17.2)
- X-ray exams for parasites include: chest x-rays for paragonimiasis, hydatid cyst, and tropical pulmonary eosinophilia
- Serologic tests are available commercially for reference labs, some from the CDC; these include schistosomiasis, strongyloidiasis, trichinosis, cysticercosis, paragonimiasis, visceral larva migrans, and echinococcosis; serology for filaria is available at NIH, other serology available in research labs or CDC (see Chap. 18 for specifics)

Therapy: Depends of etiology; if no dx is obtained in the traveler w/o sx, it is reasonable to follow and recheck in 3–12 mo; if persistent, empiric treatment for strongyloides (and other helminths) w ivermectin (200 μm/kg/d × 2) or albendazole (400 mg × 1) is reasonable; remember that despite clearance of parasitemia, eosinophilia may persist for several months after treatment

14 The Asymptomatic Traveler

Inf Dis Clin N Am 1998;12:431; Trop Med Int Health 2000;5:818

OVERVIEW

Risk of persistent or recurrent travel-related illness depends on duration and itinerary of trip, potential exposure to infectious agents (ie, recreational activity, sexual activity, etc.), and pretravel preparation. The cost/effectiveness of screening travelers for inapparent illness will vary tremendously w the individual traveler. Limited data exist on particular subsets of travelers and their risk of acquired (but inapparent) infection [ie, missionaries (Am J Trop Med 1967;16:154,161), expatriate workers (Trop Geog Med 1990:119; Lancet 1986;317:86; CID 1993;17:353), Peace Corps vounteers, immigrants (see Chapter 15). In general, significant risk from inapparent disease is rare, even in these high-risk groups. Careful questioning may define a subset of travelers who may benefit from additional studies, or, more importantly, may benefit from pretravel counseling to lower risk in the future. Particular areas of importance incl hx sexual activity (several studies document incr sex contact hx, often unprotected, in travelers); contact w fresh water in schistosomiasis endemic areas, hx needle injx/vaccinations during travel, hx of recurrent malaria or other recurrently symptomatic disease while abroad. However, in residents of developing countries for >3 mo, hx and Pe may not detect high risk. Therefore:

ASYMPTOMATIC

Screening tests of possible benefit in high-risk travelers:

- Tests for STDs in travelers w high risk (ie, unprotected intercourse, multiple partners); tests of potential (unproven) benefit incl HIV screening, chlamydia/GC, and perhaps hep B, syphilis
- PPD screening in high-risk situations (ie, prolonged residence in close contact w high-prevalence groups; ideally, a pretravel PPD w booster (2 step) can be obtained; follow-up PPD testing 3 mo or more after departure from high-risk environment
- Stool O + P or copro-antigen testing is of no clear benefit
- In highly selected situations, serologic testing for parasitic infections may have benefit, though evidence is lacking. A total eosinophil count may detect higher risk subsets of travelers; examples may include persons w hx possible schistosomiasis exposure (fresh water swimming) who may be screened w schisto FAST ELISA (CDC), if treatment planned (see 18.26); or pts w incr risk future immunosuppression and hx long-term residence w local populations in tropics might benefit from strongyloides ELISA (esp if eosinophilia) (see 18.27); pts from endemic areas for onchocerciasis w hx Calabar swellings could have filarial serology (see 18.18 and 18.19)

15 Health Screening of Immigrants and Refugees

Jama 1982;247:1303; Nejm 1988;319:918; Arch Pediatr Adolesc Med 1998;152:564
A stylized approach to the health screening of new refugees and immigrants helps ensure that undiagnosed or inadequately addressed medical conditions are identified.

PREPARATION FOR THE INITIAL HEALTH SCREENING EXAM

Arrange interpreter: If the patient has limited English proficiency, you will need an interpreter; trained medical interpreters are best but may not be an option in smaller medical centers; telephone interpreter services are second best; use a high-quality speakerphone if possible; avoid use of minors; use caution with untrained interpreters who may not respect confidentiality; many immigrant communities are microcommunities in which everybody knows everybody else; same-sex interpreters may be necessary (Jama 1995;273:724)

Tuberculosis screening: Refugees and immigrants, depending on age, usually have had a single PA chest x-ray to screen for possible active pulmonary tuberculosis before embarking for the U.S.; the interpretation of this x-ray is recorded on U.S. State Department Form OF-157; new refugees typically undergo additional tuberculosis screening by state public health departments upon

U.S. arrival; non-refugee aliens may fall outside of public health TB surveillance efforts; if not contraindicated, these patients should be screened using the purified protein derivative (PPD) tuberculin skin test (5 TU/mL, 0.1 mL intradermally); the test should be read at 72 hours; 10 mm or more of induration should prompt a referral to a state TB clinic since further laboratory work, medical exams, and medication may be covered under state Medicaid programs; prior BCG vaccine should be completely discounted

Review OF-157 and vaccine supplement, if any: Refugees and immigrants usually undergo a health-screening exam before embarking for the U.S.; depending on age, a routine chest x-ray, RPR, and HIV test may be performed; the results of this exam are summarized on the U.S. State Department Form OF-157 and vaccine supplement; this form may contain valuable health information

Preliminary lab and x-ray: If feasible, consider obtaining the following laboratory and radiology studies prior to the initial health screening; most adult refugees and immigrants will have had varicella but a history of this disease is often difficult to obtain across language barriers; a sickle prep and HIV test may also be indicated in some populations; in PPD+ individuals, AST and ALT are ordered in anticipation of starting INH prophylaxis and a urinalysis to rule out possible renal TB

- *PPD positive age 0–5*: CBC, AST, ALT, lead level, HBSAg, HBSAb, varicella titer, RPR, UA, CXR (PA & LAT), stool O + P
- *PPD positive age 6–13*: CBC, AST, ALT, HBSAg, HBSAb, varicella titer, RPR, UA, CXR (PA & LAT), stool O + P
- *PPD positive age 14+*: CBC, AST, ALT, cholesterol, HBSAg, HBSAb, varicella titer, RPR, UA, CXR (PA & LAT), stool O + P
- *PPD negative age 0–5*: CBC, lead level, HBSAg, HBSAb, varicella titer, RPR, stool O + P
- *PPD negative age 6–13*: CBC, HBSAg, HBSAb, varicella titer, RPR, stool O + P
- *PPD negative age 14+*: CBC, cholesterol, HBSAg, HBSAb, RPR, varicella titer, RPR, stool O + P

INITIAL HEALTH SCREENING

For many refugees and immigrants, the initial health-screening exam in the U.S. may be their first contact with Western health care. They may not be familiar with why certain things are done, why we ask so many questions, examine the patient and then do blood tests, x-rays, and other tests. Treatments are often expected. Patients may demand a same-sex practitioner, particularly Muslim women. (J Gen IM 1995;10:369)

History: Begin the hx/PE with information related to immigration status (example: 21 yo Vietnamese male arrived in U.S. 10/21/89, Long Beach CA. Migrated to Lowell, MA 03/07/93, Portland, ME 12/30/97). In the past medical history, specifically record any medication allergies, current medications, hospitalizations, and surgeries. Record any history of trauma, including war-related physical trauma or psychological trauma associated with war, deprivation, incarceration, or torture. Record tobacco use, alcohol use, and other substance abuse. Record availability of immunization records and current immunization status. Record hepatitis B status and TB status, if known. In the social history, record information regarding accompanying family members and/or family members with whom patient is reuniting here in U.S. Record information regarding family members who were left behind, lost to contact, or killed. Record information about refugee camp situation. Record educational level in years and whether or not patient is literate in the language spoken at home.

Physical exam: The physical exam should be thorough from head to toe and include height, weight, careful vital signs, and hearing and vision screening. Pap smear, GC, and *Chlamydia* screening should be routinely performed on the first pelvic exam. Evidence of "female circumcision" may be evident on physical exam of girls and women of East African origin (Nejm 1994;331:712).

Lab review: Review any preliminary lab data.

Assessment: Assemble a list of problems or issues needing to be addressed.

Plan: Initiate any immediately necessary treatments. Offer age-appropriate health counseling. Offer family planning and STD prevention advice. Start contraception immediately if patient desires contraception. Following appropriate informed consent, begin immunization series for all routine immunizations, assuming

that, if there is no documentation, nothing has been done.
Make any necessary referrals. Schedule patient back to complete
immunization series (usually at 2 and 6 months). Schedule patient
into routine primary health care. Do not attempt to do everything
at the first visit. It will be overwhelming for you and the patient.

Document: Carefully document what you do and give patients a card
with contact numbers for your clinic or facility in the event they
should relocate. Try to provide a record of all immunizations
administered.

TOP HEALTH CONCERNS

Bear in mind the following top health concerns as a rough guide in your
approach to refugee and immigrant patients.

Primary health and dental care: For many refugees and immigrants,
health care was something episodic in response to a problem and
even then they may not have had access to Western health care
professionals. The concept of primary, preventative health care
may be totally foreign and misunderstood. Occult disease
screening methods including serum cholesterol, cancer detection by
mammography and flexible sigmoidoscopy, etc. may be unfamiliar
approaches. A scientific understanding of diseases including germ
theory and oncogenesis may not exist. Introduce your patients
gradually to primary health care approaches through regularly
scheduled appointments. Regular dental exams are also important
and poor dental hygiene is one of the most common of all
problems encountered in refugee populations. Many refugees and
immigrants may travel home (often to show off new infants) and
should be encouraged to seek proper medical travel preparation
well in advance (West J Med 1990;153:34)

Tuberculosis: Prevalence tends to be greater in populations from
developing countries. Some patients will have been treated
overseas (often under directly observed therapy, or DOT) for
suspected active TB before being allowed to enter the U.S.

Delayed immunization: Most refugees have delayed immunization
histories. Many have no history of any immunizations. Many
Cambodian and Vietnamese refugees arriving between 1982 and
1990 came out of highly organized refugee camp settings where

immunizations were routinely administered and carefully recorded. More recent refugees from the former Yugoslavia and the African republics have no immunization records. Although polio vaccine is not recommended by the ACIP for persons over age 18, refugees and immigrants from developing countries may never have had polio immunization. Hepatitis B immunization should be strongly considered for all refugees and immigrants (Nurse Practitioner 1992;17:21)

Hepatitis B: Prevalence tends to be greater in populations from developing countries. Prevalence of serologic markers for hepatitis B may approach 80% in populations from Southeast Asia and prevalence of hepatitis B surface antigen (HBSAg) may approach 10%.

Other infectious diseases: Stool ova and parasite (O + P) screening should be considered in all patients from a tropical country and possibly others who have come out of unsanitary refugee camp situations or situations where public service infrastructure has been disrupted by war or poverty. A single O + P test, instead of three at once, may be a more practical and cost-effective approach. Depending upon the outcome of test 1, additional tests may be requested, either following treatment or to increase screening sensitivity. Persistent eosinophilia in a stool O + P negative patient may prompt additional testing for extraluminal parasites and/or empiric treatment for *Strongyloides stercoralis*. An unexplained fever in refugee and immigrant patient is malaria until proven otherwise (Nejm 1993;328:1061; Nejm 1999;340:773)

Family planning and STD prevention: Assume no prior knowledge and no knowledge of birth control options. Women may need to be interviewed without husbands present.

Post-traumatic stress disorder: Referrals to appropriate psychiatric care (Am J Psychiatry 1987;144:1567)

War-related physical impairments: Referrals to appropriate orthopedic, neurology follow-up, and rehabilitation programs.

HEALTH SCREENING

ONLINE REFERENCES AND RESOURCES

1. **Immigration definitions:** United States Immigration and Naturalization Service web site: http://www.ins.usdoj.gov/graphics/glossary.htm
2. **Vaccine informed consent documents in foreign languages:** The Immunization Action Coalition web site: http://www.immunize.org/vis/index.htm#index
3. *Core Curriculum on Tuberculosis Fourth Edition*, 2000. U.S. Department of Health and Human Services, Centers for Disease Control and Prevention, National Center for HIV, STD, and TB Prevention, Division of Tuberculosis Elimination; http://www.cdc.gov/nchstp/tb/pubs/corecurr/default.htm.

Section IV

TRAVEL-RELATED INFECTIOUS DISEASES AND OTHER AILMENTS

16 Bacteria

16.1 ANTHRAX

CID 1994;19:1009; JAMA 1999;281:1735.

Cause: *Bacillus anthracis*

Epidem: Tropical areas of So America, Haiti, Africa, Asia. 200,000 cases/yr (Wilson, 1991); animal reservoir; contact w animals or their hides is usual source; spores persist in soil for years

Risk in travelers: Very rare; contact w animal products in markets (ie, goatskin handicrafts, etc.) implicated in rare cases in travelers (Wilson, 1991); CDC reports no cases in U.S. travelers 1993–2000

Incubation period: 1–7 d

Pathophys: 3 distinct toxins, dissem from innoculation site (ie, skin, lungs, gut)

Sx: Cutaneous (90%)—papule to vesicles to ulcer w eschar in 2 d; edema out of propotion to size of lesion (often on face, neck, upper extremities); Ddx tularemia, plague, rickettsial, bact ecthyma; inhalational—flu-like illness to severe dyspnea in 2–3 d; gastrointestinal—fever, abd pain, bacteremia

Si: Skin lesions, edema, lymphadenopathy, fever, often meningismus

Crse: Variable; 10% of cutaneous lesions disseminate; higher w pulm/GI infx

Dx: Gram's stain—gram neg rods, few WBC; culture blood, eschar fluid, etc., on special media

Rx: Penicillin G (alternatives incl Cipro, doxycycline)

Prevent: Vaccination (not routinely available), but used in military and special circumstances (Jama 1999;282:2104; Mmwr 2000;49:1); postexposure prophylaxis w ciprofloxacin (500 mg q 12 hr) or amoxicillin; contact precautions

16.2 ATYPICAL MYCOBACTERIA

Cause: Atypical Mycobacterium spp. (MOTT: mycobacterium other than tuberculosis)

Epidem: Worldwide; *M. scrofulaceum* and *kansasii* etc. (MSK): Endemic in soil (*kansasii*); little person-to-person spread

M. ulcerans: Africa, Australia; causes chronic skin ulcer (Buruli ulcer)

M. marinum: worldwide; chronic granulomatous skin/soft tissue infx assoc w fresh/saltwater exp to traumatized skin, sometimes with puncture by fish spines

M. avium and *intracellulare* (MAI) ubiquitous; major problem in AIDS where is 3rd most common opportunistic infection after *Pneumocystis* and Kaposi's (Nejm 1996;335:428)

M. fortuitum and other fast growers (FG): can cause soft tissue infx after puncture wounds (Ann IM 1970;73:971); normal throat inhabitant?

Risk for travelers: Rare

Sx:

MSK: pulmonary, scrofula, skin ulcers; seen in AIDS pts (Ann IM 1991;114:861)

MU: undermined necrotic ulcers on extensor surfaces

MAI: pulmonary, especially in COPD, AIDS, and previously damaged lung but not always (Nejm 1989;321:863)

FG: pulmonary; subcutaneous abscess; corneal infection

Si: Pulmonary; nodular or ulcerative skin lesions, nodular lymphangitis

Crs:

MAI: Disseminated disease in HIV pts w CD4 count <50

FG: Spontaneous resolution w/o rx or w debridement

Cmplc:

MSK: full gamut like regular tbc; drug resistance common

FG: r/o *M. marinum*, which causes SWIMMING POOL GRANULOMA (Nejm 1997;336:1065)

Lab:

Bact: All are nicotinic acid nonproducers in contrast to *M. bovis* and *tuberculosis*. All are acid fast; grow at 25°C; are avirulent to guinea pigs; chromogen characteristics: MSK shows photochromogen; MAI, no chromogen; FG no chromogen and fast growth (2–7 d); r/o scotochromogen types, which are rarely clinically significant

Skin tests: MSK and MAI are specific and cause 2nd strength PPD to be positive

Rx: Surgery, if possible, + 2–4 drugs (Nejm 1996;335:377, 1993;329:898; Ann IM 1994;121:905) such as clarithromycin or azithromycin + ethambutol + clofazimine or rifabutin or rifampin or Cipro or amikacin; depends upon species; interferon-α may also help (Nejm 1994;330:1348)

16.3 BACILLUS CEREUS FOOD POISONING

Jama 1994;271:1074; Nejm 1978;298:143

Cause: *Bacillus cereus*

Epidem: Worldwide; commonly reported in Europe, rare in U.S.; wide variety of food types implicated w common hx of exposure to ambient temperatures for long periods after cooking

Risk for travelers: Incr risk in warm climates likely, partic where refrigeration inadequate

Pathophys: Heat-stable toxin produced in unrefrigerated rice: stays when fried and causes nausea and vomiting; a heat labile enterotoxin causes diarrhea

Incubation period: Emetic type: 1–6 hr; diarrheal type: 6–24 hr

Sx: Nausea and vomiting; or diarrhea and abdominal cramps

Si: No fever; nausea and vomiting, diarrhea

Crs: 8–10 hr for emetic type; 24–36 hr duration for diarrheal type

Cmplc: Fulminant liver failure and rhabdomyolysis (Nejm 1997;336:1142); if diarrhea, r/o clostridial or staph toxin colitis, which also lack fever

Lab:

   Bact: Dx requires isolation from foods; presence in stool is suggestive

Rx: Symptomatic

Prevent: Avoid refried rice or rice dishes (or other perishable foods) left at room temp for hrs

16.4 BACTERIAL DYSENTERY (SHIGELLOSIS)

Cause: Shigella spp (dysenteriae, flexneri, boydii, sonnei)

Epidem: Worldwide; fecal/oral especially via water supplies, bacteria die fast with drying; or person to person; increased incidence in Asia *(dysenteriae)*, also most malignant; *sonnei* most benign; infective dose low (~100 organisms) when compared w other bacterial diarrheas; causes 5–15% of diarrheal or dysenteric disease in children treated in tropical clinics

Risk for travelers: low (2–8% of traveler's diarrhea), mostly pediatric

Pathophys: Endotoxins, noninvasive so no bacteremias; superficial mucosal ulcerations, can produce DIC, hemolytic anemia, renal microangiopathy (Nejm 1978;298:926)

Incubation period: 24–72 hr

Sx: Nausea, vomiting, and severe diarrhea with cramps (75%); fever (75%); 50% of cases have both

Si: Bloody stool, watery similar to cholera

Crs: Average 2–4 d; duration ~1 wk

Cmplc: Incapacitating with low mortality, except *S. dysenteriae* often fatal; may cause hemolytic uremic syndrome (HUS); Reiter's syndrome

Lab:

> *Bact*: Gram-negative rod; stool culture; stool smear shows polys (Ann IM 1972;76:697)

Rx: Symptomatic: oral or iv lyte/fluid replacement, opiates to slow diarrhea, although theoretically could worsen by decreasing motility

> Antibiotics: ciprofloxacin (Ann IM 1992;117:727) 500 mg po bid × 5 d for *S. dysenteriae*, 1 g po × 1 ok for other species; or azithromycin 500 mg po day 1, 250 mg qd d 2–5 (Ann IM 1997;126:697); or Tm/S (Nejm 1980;303:426); ampicillin 500 mg qid, questionably effective

Prevent: Standard dietary precautions

16.5 BARTONELLOSIS (CARRION'S DISEASE, VERRUGA PERUANA)

Cause: *Bartonella bacilliformis*

Epidem: Limited to Andes Mts of Peru, Ecuador, Colombia (500–3200 m); highest risk in river valleys where sandfly vector is common, active after dusk

Risk for travelers: Rare, but recently described in Urubamba River valley, an area frequented by tourists (Am J Trop Med 1999;61:344)

Pathophys: Bacteria adhere to erythrocytes, invade endothelial cells, rbc; resulting deformity of rbc

Incubation period: 3 wk to 3 mo

Sx: Fever, ha, malaise

Si: Fever, lymphadenopathy, petechial rash (sometimes), mental status change

Crs: Resolution over wks; nodular rash of verruga peruana may develop over 1–2 mos, persist for yrs

Cmplc: CHF, pericarditis/tamponade, opportunistic infx

Lab: Coombs' neg hemolytic anemia

Dx: Blood smear shows rbc inclusions; PCR also useful

Rx: Acute phase: penicillin or choramphenicol, quinolones; chronic (verruga phase): rifampin

Prevent: Avoid sandfly bites in endemic areas w repellants, fine mesh nets; leave high-risk habitats by dusk

16.6 BITE WOUND INFECTIONS

Nejm 1985;313:991; Ann Emerg Med 1984;13:155

Cause: Anaerobes, and *Pasteurella multocida* in animal bites

Epidem: *P. multocida* is the organism in >50% of animal bite wound infections, esp from cats, which can also induce infections in scratches

Risks for travelers: Moderate in adventurous travelers (college students, etc.); 1–2% expatriates report bites per year in developing countries (Nejm 2000;342:1723)

Pathophys: Tissue damage w local infx, which then may disseminate

Sx: Localized pain, swelling, redness

Si: Cellulitis; puncture site or crush

Crs: 70% develop within 1 d, 90% in 2 d, 100% in 3 d

Cmplc: Involvement of tendon sheaths, joints, bone is problematic; rare endocarditis

Lab: Culture of purulent material often confirms Pasteurella

Rx: Prophylactic antibiotics reasonable, especially w cat bites, of which 50% get infected:
- 1st augmentin (amoxicillin and clavulinic acid); or
- 2nd penicillin; or
- 3rd tetracycline, or ampicillin, or oxacillin 500 qid × 5 d, or erythromycin, or cephalothin
- REMEMBER RABIES RISK and consider appropriate postexposure treatment

Prevent: Caution re: contact w unfamiliar dogs, cats, monkeys, etc.

16.7 BOTULISM

Ann IM 1998;129:221; Nejm 1973;289:1005

Cause: *Clostridium botulinum* (types A, B, E are the most common human pathogens)

Epidem: Worldwide; wound or food contamination; risk foods differ in different cultures (ie, in China, homemade fermented beans are source; in arctic native cultures, fermented fish are vehicle; in U.S., home canning of vegetables or fruits); heat-resistant spores contaminate:
- Canned foods or opened cans kept for days unrefrigerated (Ann IM 1996;125:558) leading to bacterial proliferation of exotoxin, which then is ingested without further heating (eg, homemade salsa, relish, canned vegetables or meats, garlic in oil, etc.)
- Wounds where bacterial proliferation and exotoxin production (80% type A, 20% type B)

Spores common in dirt and dust

Risk for travelers: Very rare

Pathophys: Exotoxin is heat-labile, extremely toxic (<1 lb could kill the world); inhibits transmitter release at all cholinergic endings; in infants and occasionally in adults (Nejm 1986;315:239) with impaired gastric acid, can generate toxin in human GI tract

Incubation period: 12 hr to several days

Sx: Mild GI sx; descending paralysis of motor and autonomic nerves starting w cranial nerves: double vision, dysphagia, dysarthria; upper respiratory tract paralysis with trouble breathing and swallowing

Si: "Myasthenia gravis that doesn't respond to edrophonium (Tensilon)" though some may a little (Ann IM 1981;95:443); flaccid paralysis

Crs: Pts can survive and recover with respirator and other supportive care for weeks to months

Cmplc: R/o myasthenia, Guillain-Barré, diphtheria, Eaton–Lambert syndrome; intoxication w organophosphates, CO, paralytic shellfish toxins (see 21.3)

Lab:

Bact: smear of food shows gram-pos bacilli; food and/or stool culture grows obligate anaerobe; extract kills mice

CSF: normal

Noninv: EMG shows low-amplitude response to nerve stimulation increased by 50/s repetitive stimulation (Nejm 1970;282:193); 15–40% false neg

Prevent: Heat all canned food prior to serving; avoid heavily fermented local foods; immunization impractical on widespread scale

Rx: Passive immunization with polyvalent horse antitoxin helps before severe sx set in, available from CDC; type-specific if possible; debride wounds; gastric lavage if food recently ingested; Supportive care, eg, respirator, etc. × weeks to months usually successful; guanidine not helpful (Nejm 1971;285:773)

16.8 BRUCELLOSIS (UNDULANT FEVER)

Medicine 1996;75:195

Cause: *Brucella melitensis* (goats), *abortus* (cattle), *suis* (pigs)

Epidem: Worldwide; Mediterranean littoral, Middle East, Latin America (Mexico, Peru, Argentina), via ingestion or contact with infected milk or meat; in rural areas; 4% of all U.S. cattle have, but marked decrease in cases in U.S. in past 50 yr

Risk for travelers: Low, but incr w ingestion of unpasteurized dairy, animal contact

Incubation period: 10 d to few mo

Pathophys: Intracellular organism causes endotoxin production; granuloma formation; diffuse systemic infestations can cause osteomyelitis

Sx:

Acute: deep bone pain; fever, sweats, malaise, headache, arthralgias (50%)

Chronic: weakness, aches, anxiety; a great mimicker of all diseases

Si:

Acute: fever, undulating to peaks in PM; deep bone pain; lymphadenopathy; splenomegaly; hepatomegaly; tenderness; arthritis; orchidoepidydimitis

Chronic: low-grade fever

Crs: Chronic, relapsing for months

Cmplc: Endocarditis, neurobrucellosis (1–5%) causes meningoencephalitis; hepatosplenic abscess

Lab:

Bact: blood and reticuloendothelial tissue grow gram-neg bacilli on culture; sens of bone marrow is 90%; ask lab to hold cultures for 4 wk

Hem: ESR low, r/o trichinosis, psittacosis, leptospirosis, CHF; mild anemia, leukopenia

Serol: hemagglutination antibody titer increased

Skin test: delayed hypersensitivity to intracutaneous antigen

Xray: Osteomyelitis

Rx: (Ann IM 1992;117:25); doxycycline 100 mg po bid + rifampin 15 mg/kg/d po × 6 wk, or streptomycin 1 gm qd × 15 d w doxy kept up for 6 wk

Prevent: Pasteurization of dairy products

16.9 CAMPYLOBACTER DIARRHEA

Ann IM 1983;98:360; 1983;99:38; Lancet 1990;336:921

Cause: *Campylobacter jejuni*

Epidem: Worldwide; accounts for 3–30% of traveler's diarrhea; esp common in winter travelers to Mexico, Morrocco, Asia (JID 1992;165:385); contaminated water, surface water, and municipal water supplies (Ann IM 1982;96:293); also may be sporadic,

foodborne, often by eggs; cattle, goats, horses, and perhaps wild
animals excrete in feces

Risk for travelers: Moderate to high (seasonal); incr risk chronic infx w
HIV; causes >30% of acute diarrhea among U.S. military in
Thailand

Incubation period: 1–7 d

Pathophys: Gut tissue invasion and exotoxin production; rare
bacteremia

Sx: Diarrhea (100%), cramps (95%), fever (80%), bloody diarrhea
(29%)

Si: Abd distension, tenderness (esp RLQ)

Crs: 20% last over 1 wk; relapses in 10%

Cmplc: Chronic colitis; Guillain-Barré syndrome (Nejm 1995;333:1374;
Ann IM 1993;118:847); r/o ulcerative colitis relapses

Lab:
   Bact: Stool culture in 10%, $CO_2 \times 48$ hr, special media

Rx: Erythromycin if sx >3 d, or azithromycin 500 mg/d for 3–5 d;
ciprofloxacin (Arch IM 1990;150:541), or other quinolone though
some drug resistance appearing to quinolones, esp in Thailand
(CID 1995;21:536)

Prevent: Proper precautions for food and water

16.10 CAT SCRATCH FEVER

Nejm 1997;337:1876, 1994;330:1509; Ann IM 1993;118:388

Cause: *Bartonella henselae* (Nejm 1994;330:509; Ann IM
1993;118:331). *Afipia felis*, a closely related organism, may be
the cause in some cases (see also trench fever, 16.48)

Epidem: Worldwide; young cats, infected for a few weeks; transmit via
bites, scratches, and fleas; 80% of cases are in pts under age 21

Risk for travelers: = domestic U.S. risk, w cat contact

Pathophys: Granuloma formation w eventual suppurative lymphadenitis

Incubation period: For initial papule, 4–8 d; for lymph nodes, 10–30 d

Sx: Bite or scratch by kitten (90% have had by hx); then papule at site
of scratch; papule at site of infection; fever (<50%), adenopathy
(40% of nodes suppurate)

Si: As above

Crs: All benign including cmplc

Cmplc: Encephalopathy/encephalitis (10%), conjunctivitis, purpura
(suppressed platelets), mesenteric adenitis, endocarditis (Ann IM
1996;125:646); hypercalcemia (Jama 1998;279:532)

   AIDS patients (Ann IM 1988;109:449) and otherwise
   immunocompromised hosts, disseminated disease:
   - BACILLARY ANGIOMATOSIS (Nejm 1997;337:1876, 1888,
     1916; 1995;332:419, 424), which looks somewhat like Kaposi's
     sarcoma, cutaneous and deep tissue infections as well as osteolytic
     bone lesions
   - PELIOSIS HEPATIS (Nejm 1992;327:1625; 1990;323:1573, 1581),
     occasionally also seen in the immunocompetent (Ann IM
     1993;118:363); see 20.11

Lab:

   CSF: protein increased; occasionally mononuclear cells in 10%
   Bact: small pleomorphic gram-neg
   Hem: elevated ESR and white count with left shift; eosinophils
   elevated modestly
   Path: biopsy shows organism with Warthin–Starry and silver stains
   Serol: Bartonella henselae titers >1/64 (84% sens, 96% specif; Nejm
   1993;329:8), from CDC, available commercially as well
   Skin test: DHS pos in 30 d, homemade from ground-up nodes; no
   longer used due to AIDS and other viral risks

Rx: None may be indicated in mild disease except aspiration of
fluctuant nodes to decrease sx of disease:
   - Erythromycin 500 mg po qid or other macrolide, esp for
     disseminated forms
   - Doxycycline 100 mg po bid, esp for disseminated forms if can't
     tolerate erythromycin
   - Ciprofloxacin 500 mg po bid (Jama 1991;265:1563)
   - Tm/S for children
   - Gentamicin iv × 5 d (West J Med 1991;154:330)
   - Ceftriaxone, cefotaxime, or amikacin (J Clin Microbiol
     1991;29:2450)

Prevent: Cat scratches (esp kittens) and flea contact

16.11 CHANCROID

Ann IM 1985;102:705; 1983;98:973
Cause: *Haemophilus ducreyi* (Ann IM 1981;95:315)
Epidem: Worldwide, but primarily in developing countries; venereally spread, ie, an STD, associated with syphilis in 15%; presence of chancroid enhances HIV transmission
Risk for travelers: Rare
Incubation period: 2–15 d
Pathophys: Skin innoc to localized pustule, regional lymphadenopathy w suppurative necrosis
Sx: Painful ulcer after 2–15 d incubation
Si: Adenopathy; tender, "dirty," necrotic ulcer(s); tender bubos (40%)
Crs: Self-limited *(usually)*
Cmplc: *Superinfection can lead to extensive soft tissue necrosis (phagedenic chancroid)*
Lab:
   Bact: culture of ulcer or lymph node aspirate positive in 70–80%; PCR test also available
Rx: (Med Let 1995;37:117)
   • 1st choice for patient and contacts: erythromycin 500 mg qid × 7 d, or ceftriaxone 250 mg im once, or azithromycin 1 g po once
   • 2nd choice: ciprofloxacin 500 mg po bid × 3 d
Prevent: Use of barrier contraceptives, abstinence, partner referral for epidemiologic treatment

16.12 CHLAMYDIAL NONSPECIFIC URETHRITIS, PROCTITIS, MUCOPURULENT CERVICITIS, PELVIC INFLAMMATORY DISEASE, TRACHOMA

Nejm 1994;330:115, Ann IM 1988;108;710; 1986;104:524
Cause: *Chlamydia trachomatis*, trachoma biovar (for LGV, see 16.25)
Epidem: Worldwide; venereal: over 50% of nonspecific urethritis episodes in males; 11% of proctitis in gay males (Nejm 1981;305:195); transmission rates males to females and vice versa nearly equal as are the asx infection rates (Jama 1996;276:1737); trachoma is major cause of blindness in Asia, Africa

Risk for travelers: Low, associ w unprotected sex; trachoma is not a concern for short-term traveler

Pathophys: Invades squamocolumnar epithelial cells; initial polymorphonuclear inflammatory response followed by lymphocytes, plasma cells, macrophages

Sx: 1/3 asx in males

Si: Urethral discharge in male; proctitis, mild in gays; cervical swab shows yellow mucopurulent discharge (14% false pos; Nejm 1984;311:1; Ann IM 1982;97:216); pharyngitis, from fellatio (Ann IM 1985;102:757)

Crs: Chronic/recurrent infx can occur; most infx self-limited

Cmplc: Epididymitis (the etiology in 1/2 the cases of epididymitis); endometritis, PID, perihepatitis like Fitzhugh–Curtis syndrome of gonorrhea; male sterility (Nejm 1983;308:502, 505; Am J Pub Hlth 1993;83:996) and female sterility (worse than gc); r/o gc and mycoplasma PID

Acute conjuctivitis in newborn (ophthalmia neonatorum) (r/o *herpes simplex* w ulcerations) from gc or chlamydia, latter more common, 5% of all deliveries; a smaller % have pneumonitis, from 1 to 60 d postpartum, average 15 d, rx w erythromycin × 14 d (Med Let 1995;35:117); in adults, inclusion conjuctivitis usually self-limited; ocular trachoma causes chronic follicular conjuctivitis, conjuctival/corneal scars

Lab:

Bact: single swab culture is 100% specif, 75% sens (Ann IM 1987;107:189); smears: males have >4 polys/hpf by urethral swab even if no discharge; females have 10^+ polys/hpf (at 1000×), 17% false pos, 10% false neg (Nejm 1984;311:1)

Path: Pap smear detection unreliable

Serol: Enzyme immunoassay method (ELISA) on secretions or urine (Jama 1993;270:2065) can be done in <30 min; 80% sens, 98% specif (Ann IM 1987;107:189); use to screen; DNA amplification assay of urine very accurate, 89% sens, 99% specif, ? availability (Nejm 1998;339:739, 768; Ann IM 1996;124:1)

Rx:

Prevent w:

• In adult, barrier methods.

• At birth, tetracycline 1% ointment × 1 (Nejm 1988;318:653), or erythromycin 0.5% ointment × 1, or silver nitrate gtts, such

antibiotic rx still misses some gc, hence there still is a 10–20%
incidence of ophthalmic disease in newborns of infected mothers
(Nejm 1989;320:769); povidone iodine 2.5% soln gtts OU is more
effective, less toxic, and cheaper (Nejm 1995;332:562)

Screen:

- All multiple partnered asx men (Jama 1996;276:1737) and
  women to reduce PID sterilization rates from 2% to 1%/yr
  (Nejm 1996;334:1362), or all women under age 25–30
  (Nejm 1998;339:739, 768; Ann IM 1998;128:277)
- All pregnant women early and at 36 wk w cultures if expected
  prevalence >7% (Ann IM 1987;107:188), or at least lower
  socioeconomic groups, and rx positives with erythromycin 500 mg
  qid × 7 d; this strategy decreases postnatal eye and lung infections,
  when given asx mothers prepartum, from infections in 50% of
  infants to 7% (Nejm 1986;314:276); for ocular trachomas, prevent
  w facial hygiene, reduction of house fly density

Rx: of active disease (Med Let 1995;37:117) by treating patient and
     partner (Med Let 1994;36:1; Nejm 1978;298:490) with:

1st:

- Azithromycin (Zithromax) 1 g po × 1 (Jama 1995;274:545; Nejm
  1992;377:921; Med Let 1991;33:119)
- Tetracycline 500 mg qid × 7 d (Ann IM 1982;97:216), 250 qid ×
  14–21 d, or doxycycline 100 bid × 7 d, or × 2–3 wk for proctitis
- Ofloxacin 300 mg po bid × 7 d
- Minocycline 100 mg po hs × 7 d (Ann IM 1993;119:16)

2nd (1st choice in pregnancy):

- Erythromycin 500 mg qid × 7 d or × 3 wk after tetracycline failure
  (Ann IM 1990;113:21), which may be due to tetracycline-resistant
  ureaplasma, for adults; nonestolated types ok in pregnancy (Med
  Let 1991;33:119); 12.5 mg/kg/d po or iv × 14 d for neonatal
  pneumonia or conjunctivitis

16.13 CHOLERA

Nejm 1985;312:343; Jama 1994;154:551

Cause: Vibrio cholerae 01, and serogroup 0139 (SE Asia)

Epidem: Worldwide in tropics; sewage in drinking water; carriers (in gallbladder) = 3–5% of world population (Ann IM 1970;72:357); primarily in Asia, So. America, and No Africa; 80 cases/yr in U.S., all but one imported (Jama 1996;276:307); many asx cases

Risk for travelers: Rare (0.001–0.01% per month); incr in cases in expatriates living in So America (CID 1996;22:1108); may be incr risk w achlorhydria, or use of drugs that block gastric acid

Pathophys: Na pump inhibition by entero/exotoxin; glucose important to that pump (Nejm 1985;312:28)

Incubation period: 12–72 hr

Sx: Diarrhea; sometimes fever

Si: "Rice water" diarrhea up to 15 L/d; "dishwater hands" from volume depletion

Crs: Benign if replace H_2O and salt iv or via NG tube

Cmplc: Mortality significant in symptomatic disease without rx; increased anion gap acidosis (Nejm 1986;315:1591)

Lab:

Bact: gram-negative rod, flagellated; culture carriers post Mg^{++} purge (30% false neg; Ann IM 1970;72:357)

Chem: stool cyclic AMP increased

Rx: (Mmwr 1991;40:562; Med Let 1991;33:107)

Acute disease:

- Oral rehydration solutions; catch up, then stool output +100 cc q 1 h (Ann IM 1975;82:101) or iv Ringer's lactate
- Antibiotics: doxycycline 300 mg po × 1 or 100 mg po bid × 3 d; or in children, Tm/S 5 mg/25 mg/kg po bid × 3 d; or ciprofloxacin

Prevent: Vaccination w killed vaccine; 0.5–1 cc × 2 then q 1 mo if heavy exposure anticipated (Ann IM 1971;74:412); 50% effective; new live attenuated oral vaccine (CVD 103 HgR and WC/rBS) more effective (Lancet 1990;335:958); neither vaccine effective against 0139 (Bengal) strain (CID 2000;31:561–565). Standard food and water precautions, especially raw seafood, tapwater in endemic areas; consider vaccination in special circumstances (see 3.5)

16.14 CLOSTRIDIUM PERFRINGENS FOOD POISONING

Nejm 1973;289:1129

Cause: *Clostridium perfringens* type A; food (food poisoning) contamination with dirt

Epidem: Worldwide (Nejm 1972;286:1026); in most soils; 8% of people carry in stool; 3rd most common type of food poisoning after staph and salmonella; vehicle is usually meat dish stored for long period at ambient temp after cooking; type C causes life-threatening enteritis in malnourished groups, especially in New Guinea highlands (pig-bel) but also in refugee camps, etc.

Risk for travelers: Low, but incr if cooked meats not served hot

Pathophys: Exotoxin produced in food before or rarely after ingestion causing watery diarrhea via Na pump effects. May act as superantigen that releases inflammatory mediators

Sx: 12 h incubation period, then diarrhea without vomiting; no fever

Si: Usually none

Crs: Mild, only 1% call doctor; lasts 12 hr

Cmplc: R/o other diarrheal illnesses

Lab:

   Bact: smear shows large gram-pos sporulating bacilli, which in culture produce lecithinase and CO_2

Rx: Fluid replacement oral or iv

Prevent: Eat cooked foods served hot; avoid storage of cooked meats at room temp

16.15 DIPHTHERIA (MEMBRANOUS CROUP)

Ann IM 1989;111:71; Nejm 1988;318:12, 41

Cause: *Corynebacterium diphtheriae, gravis* and *mitis* strains lysogenic for a specific phage (other species are opportunistics in debilitated patients) (Ann IM 1969;70:919)

Epidem: Worldwide; epidemically present in U.S. still, and resurging in Russia and former Soviet Union states (MMWR 1996;45:693); immunization of >50% of population begins to decrease incidence; peak incidence at age 15–39 yr; female/male: 2:1; Seattle epidemic

(>1100 cases) in alcoholics (Ann IM 1989;111:71); human carriers are reservoirs; acutely ill patients are communicable only ~2 wk; skin lesions can also be both portal of entry and source of carrier state (Nejm 1969;280:135)

Risk for travelers: Rare, but may have significant local risk during regional epidemics in adults w remote vaccination hx; considered a risk in E Europe, Russia: cutaneous diphtheria also reported in travelers to developing countries of Asia, Latin America, Africa (Travel Medicine 1989; 389)

Incubation period: 2–5 d

Pathophys: Exotoxin produced by phage hits conducting cells, eg, heart and nerves; resulting anatomic changes in heart increase incidence of arrhythmias and failure years later; *gravis* strain causes more lymphadenopathy, especially in pharynx, and hits heart more often

Sx: Weakness, slight sore throat (90%), low-grade fever (85%), dysphagia and nausea (25%), ha (18%); skin ulcer

Si:
- Fever
- Membrane: exudate flows over tonsils where thickens in 2–3 d to classic fibrin pharyngeal waxy material, blue-white bleeds when peel, but has minimal inflammation
- Edema of neck (18%)
- Conjunctivitis; infected skin lesions (nonhealing; r/o strep ecthyma, other)

Crs: Mortality 5–10% w rx; higher w laryngeal disease

Cmplc:
- Airway obstruction, especially with *mitis* strain
- Cardiac arrhythmias and myocarditis especially with *gravis* strain; ECG abnormal in 65%; 10% fatality rate from cardiac arrest
- Neuropathies: peripheral (15%); rarely palatal motor impairment in first days of illness; cranial nerves III, VI, VII, IX, and X motor in 2–3 wk; Guillain-Barré rarely months later
- R/o mononucleosis, which can mimic membrane (also seen w pharyngeal anthrax)

Lab:

Bact: smear shows club-shaped, nonmotile gram-pos bacilli, close to actinomycetes; nasopharyngeal swab culture on Loeffler's slant can detect within 12 hr if holding rx; if already treated with penicillin, may grow in 1 wk on tellurite slant, sharply selective

Prevent: Active immunization of infants with toxoid in DPT 4-shot series, booster at school age, or over age 7 with 3-shot dT series; 80% of U.S. population now immunized; no deaths in patients with at least 1 immunization; q 10 yr thereafter with tetanus as dT (rv CDC-Ann IM 1985;103:896); some now argue that is unnecessary to boost adults (Lancet 1985;1:1089), but outbreak in Russia provides contrary evidence

Carrier state: penicillin as Bicillin × 1, or erythromycin (resistance developed in Seattle) 250 mg qid × 7 d (89% effective), or clindamycin 150 mg qid × 7 d

Active disease: penicillin or erythromycin (resistance developed in Seattle), of questionable help, antitoxin ineffective if given >48 h after onset and probably not worth complication risk anyway but can be done w 50,000 U antitoxin for acute *gravis* in first 24 hr and repeated in 24 h × 1

16.16 E. COLI (ENTEROPATHOGENIC, ENTEROAGGREGATIVE, ENTEROADHERENT) DIARRHEA

Cause: Toxin-producing types like O157:H7 (Nejm 1995;333:364; Ann IM 1988;109:705)

Epidem: EPEC are a major cause of epidemic diarrhea in children in developing countries; EHEC are zoonotic strains assoc w cattle, other animals, ie, O157:H7 type (Ann IM 1995;123:698) in hamburger (Jama 1984;272:1349), drinking water, and swimming lakes (Nejm 1994;331:579); most common cause of infectious bloody diarrhea in U.S.

Risk in travelers: Low

Incubation period: 2–6 d

Pathophys: Colonic wall invasion and toxin production causes bloody mucus, like shigella

Sx: Bloody mucus, or watery diarrhea w fever in most, pain

Si: Low-grade fever, fecal leukocytes present, initial watery stool becomes bloody

Crs: self-limited for most, but causes some fatalities

Cmplc: Hemolytic/uremic syndrome (in 10%; Jama 1994;272:1349; Nejm 1987;317:1496) or TTP, r/o other GI infections

Lab:
  Bact: stool smear shows polys; if polys, culture for pathogens on
    sorbitol–MacConkey agar and do O157 antiserum test of cultured
    E. coli (Nejm 1995;333:364); stool toxin titers
Rx: Rehydration and supportive care
Prevent: Food and water precautions

16.17 EHRLICHIOSIS

Jama 1996;275:199(HGE); Mmwr 1996;45:798 (HME), 1995;44:593;
  Ann IM 1994;120:730, 736; Nejm 1993;329:1164
Cause: (Nejm 1996;334:209) *Ehrlichia sennetsu* and *chaffeensis*
  (human monocytic ehrlichiosis) (HME) and unnamed sp
  (human granulocytic ehrlichiosis) (HGE)
Epidem: North America, Europe, E Asia (*E. sennetsu*); tick-borne
  (Ixodes scapularis, I. ricinus and *Amblyomma americanum)*,
  common in animals; two types: HME in Southeast Asia (where
  causes a mononucleosis-like, Sennetsu fever), now >300 cases in
  southern and central U.S. from Lone Star ticks, eg, Tennessee golf
  course epidemic (Nejm 1995;333:420); and HGE
  in midwestern and northeastern U.S. (Ann IM 1996;125:904;
  1995;123:277; Jama 1994;272:212) from deer ticks
Risk for travelers: Low, HGE assoc w deer/sheep tick contact in U.S.
  and Europe
Pathophys: Intracellular in polys or monocytes, si and sx same in both
  types
Incubation period: 10 d
Sx: Acute self-limited febrile illness, headache, malaise, chills, nausea
  and vomiting
Si: Fever; occasionally cough; arthralgias; confusion; macular rash
  (HME—30%)
Crs: Fatalities among the elderly age >60 yr
Cmplc: Pericarditis (Nejm 1996;334:213); meningoencephalitis (HME);
  perinatal transmission to newborn (Nejm 1998;339:375); r/o
  RMSF and concomitant or distinct Lyme disease or babesiosis
  (Nejm 1997;336:15, Jama 1996;275:1657); see 16.24, 16.39
Lab:
  Chem: LFTs elevated (90%)

Hem: CBC shows pancytopenia, especially thrombocytopenia, and diagnostic mulberry-like inclusions in polys (morulae) (80%) (Nejm 1995;332:1417) in HGE, rarely seen in HME type

Serol: diagnostic IFA acute (often neg) and convalescent titers; PCR whole blood w sens 50–80%

Rx: Doxycycline or other tetracycline; rifampin may have role in pregnancy

Prevent: Insect repellent and other antitick measures

16.18 GONORRHEA (GC)

Cause: *Neisseria gonorrhoeae*

Epidem: Worldwide; venereal; common; bacteremia associated with deficient complement factors, eg, C_5', C_6', C_7', C_8' (Ann IM 1983;99:35); coincident *Chlamydia* infection in 15% male heterosexuals, 25% females (Nejm 1984;310:545)

Risk for travlelers: Low, assoc w unprotected sex; antimicrobial resistant gc prevalent in Africa, Asia (Sex Transm Dis 1997;24:32)

Incubation period: 24 hr to 14 d

Pathophys: Infects mucous membrancs of GU tract (Nejm 1985;312:1683); igA protease on surface distinguished infectious *Neisseria* from commensals (Nejm 1978;299:973) as do pili; septicemia more commonly with strains with fewer GU sx, leading to rash, polyarthralgias with negative joint taps (an immune complex disease; Ann IM 1978;89:28); later one joint may evolve to a single hot infected joint (Nejm 1968;279:234)

Sx: Male: urethral discharge, but 2/3 asx (Nejm 1974;290:117); anal infections, more often asx (Ann IM 1977;86:340); pharyngitis (Nejm 1973;288:181)

Female: Bartholin cyst (80% acute Bartholin's gland cyst infections are due to gc); vaginal discharge, dysuria, pelvic inflammatory disease, pain typically occurring with menses or pregnancy, abnormal menstrual bleeding due to endometritis

Si: Urethral, anal or pharyngeal discharge; in female, abdominal distension, "chandelier sign" (severe pain w cervical motion), pus in cervix

Crs: 2–7$^+$ d latent period

Cmplc:
- Bacteremia with purpuric or vesicular pustule on broad erythematous base or later, hemorrhagic bullae
- Endocarditis, 80% have arthritis too; with monoarticular arthritis, 3% will have endocarditis
- FITZHUGH–CURTIS SYNDROME, hepatic capsule inflammation (Nejm 1970;282:1082)
- Polyarthritis and tenosynovitis (rv of all septic arthritis; Nejm 1985;312:764)
- R/o *Trichomonas*, *Candida*, *Chlamydia* (Nejm 1974;291:1175), syphilis, Reiter's, appendicitis in female

Lab:
> *Bact*: Gram's stain, in male 1st, culture only if unclear on Gram's stain; in female, smear of cleanly wiped cervix to look for >3 polys/hpf with intracellular gram-negative cocci, has a 67% sensitivity, 98% specificity
>
> *Culture*: in male only if unclear on smear; reculture all after rx and recheck VDRL if negative first time; *penicillinase-producing* strains now in U.S.
>
> *Serol*: Screen for associated complement deficiencies with CH_{50} level (Nejm 1983;308:1138)

Rx: (Med Let 1995;37:117; 1994;36:1) general rules: regimens now must be good vs *penicillinase*-producing organisms; 1st-generation cephalothins and phenoxymethyl penicillin are ineffective; tetracycline inadequate for gc but treat all with it at 500 mg qid × 7 d or doxycycline 100 mg bid to get *Chlamydia*

1st:
- Ceftriaxone 125–250 mg im × 1 ($10); gets syphilis, and both pharyngeal and resistant gc; or
- Cefixime 400 mg po × 1 ($5); or
- Cefpodoxime 200 mg po × 1 ($3) (Med Let 1992;34:107)
- Ciprofloxacin 500 mg po × 1; no good vs syphilis; resistance appearing (Ann IM 1996;125:465), esp in Philippines, Asia
- Ofloxacin 400 mg po × 1

2nd:
- Spectinomycin 2 g im × 1; if penicillin allergy; no good vs syphilis or vs gc pharyngitis, resistance developing in Army where used as first drug in Korea (Nejm 1987;317:272)

Cmplc: (Mmwr 1993;42:STD supplement:1) arthritis and/or septicemia, hospitalize and tap joint, irrigate it if worsens;

10 million U aqueous penicillin until afebrile × 3 d then 7 d
cefoxitin 1 g qid iv, or spectinomycin 2 g bid im

Prevent: Barrier contraceptives; avoid infected partners; preventive
tetracycline, in neonates, 1% ointment once, or erythromycin;
are better than AgNO₃ (Nejm 1988;318:657)

16.19 GRANULOMA INGUINALE

Ann IM 1985;102:705

Cause: *Calymmatobacterium granulomatis*

Epidem: Common in SE India, Papua NG, No Australia, parts of Brazil;
venereally spread, ie, an STD; highest rates in low-income areas

Risk in travelers: Very rare (Fewer than 30 cases/yr dx in U.S., most in
immigrants)

Incubation period: 1–4 wk for initial lesion; range up to several mo

Pathophys: Tissue infiltration w inflamm cells; large cells w inclusions
= Donovan bodies

Sx: Painless ulcer

Si: Genital papule, inguinal nodes; skin breaks down into granulation
tissue

Crs: Long term even with rx

Cmplc: Scar formation; secondary lymphedema of external genitalia

Lab:
 Path: biopsy shows diagnostic intracellular organisms, called
Donovan bodies

Rx: (Med Let 1994;36:1); 1st tetracycline; 2nd streptomycin

Prevent: Barrier contraceptives may not suffice; avoid contact w infected
person

16.20 LEGIONNAIRES' DISEASE (LEGIONELLOSIS)

Nejm 1997;337:682; J Inf Dis 1992;165:736

Cause: *Legionella pneumophilia*, etc. (Ann IM 1980;93:366)

Epidem: Worldwide; travel outbreaks reported in cruise ships
(Lancet 1996;347:494); airborne or drinking water borne
(Nejm 1992;326:151); epidemic and endemic; male > female;

summer/fall peaks; many unrecognized cases, 5% of all community-acquired pneumonias; spread by air conditioner systems (Nejm 1980;302:365); increased incidence in patients on dialysis, with DM, COPD, over age 50, on chemotherapy

Risk for travelers: Rare, though prob underdiagnosed as in U.S.; more likely in areas with developed water systems that aerosolize water (ie, cooling towers, hot water showers, etc.); outbreaks have been reported in several European resort hotels (Lancet 2000;356:177); assoc w whirlpool spa, cruise ships (CID 1999;28:33)

Incubation period: 2–10 d

Pathophys: Virulent intra-cellular bacteria (cell-mediated immunity important)

Sx: *Diarrhea (2/3); cough without sputum, pleurisy, ha, recurrent rigors; r/o mycoplasma and psittacosis

Si: *Pneumonitis, *fever, slow pulse, confusion, wound infections (Ann IM 1982;96:173)

Crs: High fatality rate if immunocompromised

Lab:

Bact: sputum Gram's stain shows polys without bugs; gram-neg rod in CYE culture, will not stain in tissue; fluorescent antibody stains of transtracheal aspirate or sputum, pos in 26% (Ann IM 1979;90:1) to 68% (Am J Med 2001;110:42); culture requires special media, very fastidious

Chem: LFTs increased (1/2); Na <130 (2/3)

Hem: ESR increased (1/3); polys increased (2/3) with left shift

Serol: titer >1/250 IgG and IgM

Urine: 3^+ protein (20%), RBCs; urine antigen by RIA or ELISA, 80% sens, 100% specif; is the clinically most useful test (Am J Med 2001;110:41)

Xray: Chest shows bilat pneumonia, 1/3 w pleural effusion

Rx: (Nejm 1998;129:328)

- Azithromycin, clarithromycin, or erythromycin × 10–14 d
- Ciprofloxacin 400 mg iv q 8 h or 750 mg po bid, or newer fluoroquinolone
- Tetracycline, but less effective

---

* Most important findings to dx

16.21 LEPROSY

Lancet 1999;353:655; CID 2001;32:930

Cause: *Mycobacterium leprae*

Epidem: Africa, India, SE Asia, Latin America; unknown mode of transmission, seems to require prolonged (>1 mo) exposure, probably skin and nasal discharge; 3–5 yr incubation; tuberculoid type is not infectious (Ann IM 1978;88:538); reservoir is armadillo (No America), primates; 15 million in world; especially children and young adults

Risk to travelers: Very rare to nonexistent; may occur in particular refugee groups to developed countries from endemic areas; 85% of detected cases in U.S. are in immigrants

Pathophys:

- Lepromatous type like sarcoid and Hodgkin's, involves impaired delayed hypersensitivity; granuloma formation leads to nerve compression? IgG and IgA increased while IgM normal (Ann IM 1969;70:295; Nejm 1968;278:298); T lymphs in lesions are all suppressor cells

- Tuberculoid type, in patients with strong response; all T cells in lesions are helper cells (Nejm 1982;307:1593)

- Both types infect colder tissues, hence hands, feet, ears, nose, peripheral nerves

Incubation period: 3 mo-40 yr (average 2–4 yr)

Sx: Years incubation period; eczematous rash; numbness (85%) anesthetic patch

Si: Lepromatous to tuberculoid spectrum: nodular accumulations in skin, mucous membranes, and other organs, especially on face, organisms are in these "globi"; to thickened peripheral nerves; to decreased sensation in extremities leading to mutilation and loss, pain and temperature sensation diminished; absent wheal and flare response; vitiligo; also diffuse skin infiltration, or plaques

Crs: chronic, relapsing

Cmplc: Arthritis, septic with bacteria in joint histiocytes (Nejm 1973;289:1410); secondary amyloid; ERYTHEMA NODOSUM LEPROSUM w painful skin nodules, fever, wasting, rx w thalidomide (Med Let 1996;38:15); neuritis, nephritis may follow rx

Lab:

Bact: Slit skin smears—AFB-positive smears of globi as well as blood and buffy coat since bacteria both free and in WBCs in lepromatous type, decrease in numbers correlates with rx over months, average rx duration = 105 mo (Nejm 1972;287:159); and of marrow histiocytes (Nejm 1979;300:834)

Path: skin bx of globi and/or nerve bx show epithelioid cell collections without distinct tubercles; nerves surrounded by microscopic tubercles

Serol: VDRL, cryoglobulin, rheumatoid factor often pos in lepromatous, not tuberculoid types

Prevent: w BCG immunization?, questionable results (Ann IM 1978;88:538); isolation unnecessary

Rx: WHO recc. depends on stage of disease, triple rx w clofazimine (Med Let 1987;29:77) 50–100 mg po qd, + sulfones, eg, DDS (Dapsone = diaminodiphenylsulfone), + rifampin; or combinations of minocycline, clarithromycin, ofloxacin, and augmentin; may make noninfectious in weeks (Ann IM 1976;85:82) to 3 mo; 2+ yr course, longer with lepromatous type

16.22 LEPTOSPIROSIS (WEIL'S DISEASE)

Nejm 1984;310:524; Ann IM 1973;79:167

Cause: *Leptospira* sp (many)

Epidem: Worldwide, esp tropics; outbreaks may occur w flooding (JID 1998; 178:1457); usually in young adults in warm seasons, from contact with or ingestion of water contaminated with animal urine or directly with the animals themselves: dogs, rats (causing urban epidemic foci; Ann IM 1996;125:794), cattle, pigs, frogs, squirrels, other wild animals, etc.

Risk for travelers: Low, but recent outbreak in "ecochallenge"; incr risk w adventure or ecotourism inv extensive water contact; 1/3 of kayakers on Costa Rican river trip infected (Mmwr 1996;46:557)

Pathophys: Biphasic illness; Weil's disease is the 2nd, immune phase with rash, hepatitis, renal failure, myocarditis, uveitis

Incubation period: 2–26 d (average = 10 d)

Sx: Abrupt onset of "flu syndrome"; malaise; headache often severe; fever; nausea, vomiting, diarrhea (50%); dry cough; myalgias; jaundice though not always clinical

Si: Icterus, fever, purpura and other rashes, tender organomegaly, conjunctivitis, severe muscle tenderness; r/o dengue, adenovirus, toxic shock, rubella, rubeola, Kawasaki's

Crs: 2–5% mortality without rx, rest eventually resolve

Cmplc: Weil's disease or syndrome: elevated bilirubin and BUN, anemia, uveitis, hemorrhages, aseptic meningitis with mental status changes; myocarditis, renal failure, hepatic failure, meningitis

Lab:

Bact: Culture of urine up to 6–8 wk after onset, or acute CSF or blood on special media from CDC at 30°C × 6 wk; or guinea pig (not rodent) injection causes icterus in 3–12 d

Chem: CPK, bilirubin, BUN (25%), LFTs all increased

CSF: Aseptic meningitis pattern

Hem: ESR low, r/o brucellosis, trichinosis, psittacosis

Urine: RBCs

Serol: MAT (CDC) is gold standard; newer IHA and Eliza–IgM helpful; sensitivity may vary w geography

Rx: (Lancet 1988;1:433), 1st tetracycline 2–4 g qd, or doxycycline as below; 2nd, penicillin

Prevent: w doxycyline 100 mg po bid × 1 wk (Ann IM 1984;100:696; Nejm 1984;310:497) if likely exposed, or doxycycline 100 mg per wk for high-risk travel

16.23 LISTERIAL INFECTIONS

Nejm 1996;334:770

Cause: Listeria spp

Epidem: Worldwide; present in most soils, animal GI tracts, and raw milk from infected cows, though it can occur even if pasteurized (Nejm 1997;336:100; 1985;312:404) or cheese (Mexican cheese epidemic in Calif; Nejm 1988;319:823); increased in pregnant women, elderly, neonates (Nejm 1971;285:599), and immunocompromised (Ann IM 1992;117:466)

Risk in travelers: Rare (similar to nontravelers), though risk increased w regular dietary use of unpast dairy

Incubation period: 2 d to 2 wk

Pathophys: Intracellular pathogenesis, usually picked up by gut macrophages and spread from there

Sx: Sepsis, meningitis, vertigo

Si: Sepsis, meningitis especially in children < age 6 mo (p54); rhomboencephalitis w ataxia, brainstem sx

Crs: Often prolonged; req several wks of antibiotics

Cmplc: Meningitis, rhomboencephalitis, sepsis, spontaneous abortion

Lab: Blood cx often positive (may be initially mistaken by lab for diphtheroids)

CSF: Gram-positive rods, tumbling motility; often <80% polys

Rx: Ampicillin first choice; Tm/S a second choice or used w ampicillin

Prevent: Pastuerized dairy products

16.24 LYME DISEASE

Nejm 1993;329:936; 1989;320:133; 2001;345:115

Cause: *Borrelia burgdorferi* spread by *Ixodes scapularis* or *pacificus* tick bite (same tick also spreads babesiosis, human granulocytic ehrlichiosis and patients may get both; Ann IM 1985;103:374) in No America, *Ixodes ricinus* carries similar organisms (w addition of tickborne encephalitis virus) in Europe, *I. persulcatus* in Asia

Epidem: Northern temp zones of No America and Eurasia; deer tick (U.S.) and sheep tick (Europe), infests small rodents, which are reservoir host for *B. burgdorferi*; most common tickborne spirochetal disease in U.S.; attack rates up to 66% of people living in a highly endemic area over 7 yr (Nejm 1989;320:133); annual incidence = 20–80/100,000/yr; also common in No Europe (Nejm 1995;333:1319)

Risk for travelers: Low, but focally moderate to high risk in individuals w exposure to ticks in highly endemic sites (esp coastal islands) in northeastern U.S., or hikers in European forested areas during summer months

Pathophys: Sometimes an immune complex disease, but organisms now identified in joints most of the time (Nejm 1994;330:229); clinical syndromes like primary, secondary, and tertiary syphilis; but much overlap between stage 1 and 2 sx complexes

Incubation period: 3–30 d post bite for early disease; later stages may present mos later

Sx: (Nejm 1991;325:159) Tick bites usually painless (should remove w tweezers) hx in 30% (Nejm 1995;333:1319); disease rare if tick on <24 hr, usually takes 72 hr and most ticks associated w disease have stayed on a week (Nejm 1992;327:543)

- Stage 1: EM rash plus systemic sx in 1/2 (arthralgias (98%), malaise (80%), headache (64%), fever (60%), stiff neck), circular or oval expanding macular rash erythema migrans (EM) in 77% (Nejm 1995;333:1319); rash appears days to weeks after tick bite; nearly always 5 cm or more in diameter at onset, w median size 15 cm in some series

- Stage 2: neurologic (headache, paresthesias, focal weakness) and cardiac (dizziness, syncope)

- Stage 3: arthritis (swollen large joint—usually asymmetric); chronic neurologic changes

Si:

- Stage 1: fever, lymphadenopathy; and erythema migrans, a warm flat lesion around bite, median diam = 15 cm (pictures; Ann IM 1991;114:490; 1983;99:76) present in 60–80%; can have vesicular center (5%), or multiple same sized lesions (10%); unlike ringworm, not scaly; may have homogeneous erythema or target lesions

- Stage 2: neurologic: lymphocytic meningitis (15%) and meningoencephalitis, peripheral motor or sensory neuropathies, facial nerve palsies including Bell's palsy; and/or cardiac: myocarditis (8%), similar rheumatic fever with heart block but valve disease rare or never; sometimes heart block is only sx, no fever or even malaise; usually transient, ~6 wk after primary infection

- Stage 3: recurrent asymmetric oligoarticular arthritis at 1st, then 1–2 large joints; onset up to 4–6 mo after skin rash with decreasing recurrences over years (Ann IM 1987;107:725); late keratitis (Nejm 1991;325:159)

Crs: Stage 1 lasts 3–4 wk; Sx and si of stages 2 and 3 may be chronic and recurrent over mo–yr; Even after rx, esp if given >3 mo after sx, residual arthralgias, fatigue, memory problems may persist (Ann IM 1994;121:560) but overall response to Rx is good; very benign crs in children (Nejm 1996;335:1270)

Cmplc: Neurologic (Nejm 1990;323:1438): encephalopathy is
uncommon; also chronic polyneuropathy and leukoencephalitis;
r/o Ehrlichiosis (16.17), babesiosis (18.7) as separate or
concomitant infection
(Nejm 1997;337:27; Jama 1996;275:1657)

Lab:

Hem: ESR >20 mm/h (53%), crit >37% (88%), WBC <10,000 (92%)

Path: Pos silver stain or culture of rash edge for organisms in 86%
(Jama 1992;268:1311)

Serol: (Ann IM 1997;127:1109) need reliable lab; IgM and IgG
ELISA titer increased (Nejm 1983;308:733) and pos Western blot;
false positives, most in low-prevalence populations, in syphilis, and
SBE (Ann IM 1993;119:1079); = 5%, false neg especially in late
stages (Ann IM 1987;107:730), seen if early po antibiotic rx or
early in crs, or w some labs, which run 10–50% false neg and up
to 25% false pos (Jama 1992;268:891)

Synovial fluid: Organisms usually present by PCR (Nejm
1994;330:229)

Rx: (Med Let 1997;39:47, Jama 1995;274:66; Ann IM 1991;111:472)

- Prevent w permethrin (Nix) rx of clothing and DEET at 30–75$^+$%
concentration (Med Let 1989;31:46); remove ticks within 24 hr;
vaccinate w Osp-A antigen 75–95% effective after 3-shot series
(Nejm 1998;339:209, 216, 263)

- Prophylactic rx after tick bite may be useful, perhaps 2 doses
(100 mg) of doxycycline if fully engorged deer tick in high-
prevalence area (Med Let 1992;34:95; Nejm 2001;345)

- Rx stage 1 (Med Let 1989;31:57): to decrease post-rash arthritis
and illness (Ann IM 1983;99:22) with 1st, tetracycline 250 mg qid
or doxycycline 100 mg bid × 21 d; or amoxicillin 250–500 mg po
tid × 21 d; or 2nd, azithromycin 500 mg/d × 5 d, or cefuroxime 500
mg po bid × 21 d (Ann IM 1992;117:273)

- Stages 2 and 3: doxycycline 200 mg po bid or amoxicillin as above
(Nejm 1994;330:229) or ceftriaxone 2 gm iv/im × 14–21 d
especially if recurrent arthritis or cardiac/neurologic findings, only
1/13 failures (Nejm 1988;319:1661); or penicillin G 20 million U
qd iv × 10–21 d for cardiac, or neurologic abnormalities and/or
meningitis (Ann IM 1983;99:767); avoid intraarticular steroids
(Nejm 1985;312:869)

- Acute non-meningitis disseminated disease: doxycycline 100 mg
po bid × 21 d, equally effective as ceftriaxone 2 gm im qd × 14 d

(Nejm 1997;337:289)
- Heart block: antibiotics and temporary pacer (Ann IM 1989;110:339)
- Chronic encephalopathy: 60–85% improve with ceftriaxone rx given, even after several years
- Pos titers and chronic fatigue/fibromyalgia syndrome, no rx (Ann IM 1993;119:503, 518)

16.25 LYMPHOGRANULOMA VENEREUM

Ann IM 1983;98:973; Nejm 1978;298:494

Cause: *Chlamydia trachomatis,* immuno type L

Epidem: Worldwide; endemic in many developing countries; venereally spread; highest incidence in gay males; male/female: 20:1

Risk for travelers: Very low, assoc w unprotected sex, contact w prostitutes

Pathophys: Granulomatous response w stellate microabcess formation

Incubation period: Few days to 1 mo

Sx: Painless papule (30%); bubo (70%); long incubation period

Si: Adenopathy, local and distant; fever; erythema nodosum; ulcerative proctitis, in gays (Nejm 1981;305:195)

Crs: Gradual resolution over wks/mos; 20% relapse w/o Rx

Cmplc: Rectal stricture; cancer develops in 2%

Lab: Review of dx tests (Nejm 1983;308:1563)
  Bact: culture possible and quite easy
  Serol: comp-fix antibody pos (>1/16) in 60%, r/o psittacosis
  Skin test: pos (>6 mm at 48 hr)

Rx: (Med Let 1995;37:117); tetracycline × 21 d, often must repeat × 1–2; or erythromycin 500 mg qid × 21 d

Prevent: Barrier contraceptives may not be adequate; avoid sexual contact w inf person

16.26 MELIOIDOSIS

Cause: *Pseudomonas pseudomallei*

Epidem: Ubiquitous bacteria of soil, but esp common cause of human disease in SE Asia, No Australia; assoc w rice paddies; contracted by inhalation/ingestion or possible abrasion; in No Thailand, accounts for 20% of admits for sepsis (J Infect Dis 1989;159:890)

Risk for travelers: Low; most cases in U.S. have been in immigrants from Asia; also in returning military personnel or others w extensive field exposure; est 300 cases dx in U.S. soldiers in Vietnam; 5% seropositive (Wilson, 1991); seroprevalence 2% in U.S. diplomats in Thailand (J Travel Med 2001;8:146)

Incubation period: 2 d to mos; latent period of up to 20 yr

Sx: Acute: localized wound infx, pneumonia, sepsis
Indolent: resp infx like tbc

Si: Acute: pustular/necrotic skin lesions; pneumonia

Crse: Fulminant or indolent (Ddx tbc)

Lab: Gram-neg bacilli w "safety pin" bipolar staining pattern w methylene blue; grows on routine media

Rx: TCN (but resistant strains reported in Thailand), piperacillin, imipenem, 3rd-gen ceph; combination rx w 2 drugs may be necessary in severe cases

16.27 MENINGOCOCCAL MENINGITIS

Nejm 2001;344:1378; 1992;327:864; Ann IM 1990;112:610; 1985;102:229

Cause: (Nejm 1997;337:970) adult meningitis:
- Age 20–60: 1st pneumococcus, 2nd *Neisseria meningitidis* (serogroup Y > C > B > A), 3rd *Haemophilus influenzae*, 4th *Listeria*
- Age 60+: 1st pneumococcus, 2nd *Listeria*, 3rd others

Epidem: Worldwide; seasonal epidemics in SubSaharan Africa (meningitis belt-see Fig. 3.5); also outbreaks in pilgrims in Hajj in Saudi Arabia (Jama 1988;260:2686); serogroup A in epidemics in developing countries, rare in U.S.; groups B and C are sporadic and in epidemics in U.S. (Jama 1995;273:383, 390)

From respiratory tract of carriers (<3% of general population) or patients with meningococcal pneumonitis (Ann IM 1979;91:7); increased after influenza infection (Nejm 1972;287:5); bacteremia recurs in patients with complement deficiencies of C_6', C_7', or C_8'; (40% of all adult meningitis is nosocomial, often gram negatives, although meningococcal never is)

Risk in travelers: Increased (but rare) in visitors to SubSaharan Africa (vaccination recommended); pilgrims traveling to Hadj in Saudi Arabia (Mmwr 2001;50:97); also during outbreaks in other countries (see CDC Blue sheet)

Incubation period: 2–10 d

Pathophys: IgA protease on surface distinguishes infectious from commensal meningococcus (Nejm 1992;327:864)

URI leads to bacteremia 1st, then

- Metastatic infections of meninges, eye, pericardium, joints, and/or cardiac valves
- Shwartzman phenomena
- Immune complex arthritis without permanent damage

Sx: Fever, unusual changed affect/mental status (85%), stiff neck

Si: Fever >100°F (95%), stiff neck (88%), petechial rash with central focal necrosis (66%) (purpura fulminans pictures; Nejm 1996;334:1709), focal neurologic deficits (28%), seizures (23%); occasionally meningococcal pneumonia alone (Ann IM 1975;82:493)

Crs: Without rx, death in hrs; w rx, 25% mortality (in pneumococcal meningitis, mortality higher and morbidity >50%)

Cmplc:

- CNS thrombophlebitis with focal seizures and deficits, CN neuropathies (Nejm 1972;286:882), communicating hydrocephalus
- Myocarditis in 75% at postmortem, 20% have aseptic pericardial effusions (Ann IM 1971;74:212)
- Adrenal hemorrhage and insufficiency (Waterhouse–Friderichsen syndrome)
- Chronic bacteremia without CNS involvement, fever, or rash

Lab:

Bact: CSF has >10 white cells/mm^3, usually (87%) >200, mostly polys; glucose <40 mg % (50%); protein >45 mg % (96%), usually >100 mg %; Gram's stain shows intracellular gram-neg diplococci; culture best in 10% CO_2; blood cultures

Xray: CT scan if focal si before LP, but START ANTIBIOTICS 1ST

Prevent: In epidemic or in endemic areas by:

- Decreasing intimate contact
- Immunizing with polysaccharide antigen sc, type-specific, 85% effective vs type C or A (Ann IM 1978;89:949; Nejm 1977;297:686), others report in epidemic 67% effective under age 5, 50% under age 18, and 20% under age 30 (Jama 1998;279:435);

or w oligosaccharide-protein conjugate vaccine (like Hib vaccine for H. flu), more effective in infants (Jama 1996;275:1499)
- Administering prophylactic antibiotics (Nejm 1982;307:1266) to family, day care companions, and close friends, not school or hospital personnel unless 2 cases occur in a school (Jama 1997;277:389): rifampin 600 mg po qid × 2 d

Rx:
- Acute disease: penicillin 24 million U iv qd in q 2 h bolus × 1 d then q 4 h for meningococcal type and covers 64% of pneumococcus as well (Nejm 1997;337:970); does not eliminate carrier state; also drug of choice in head trauma since most likely organism is pneumococcus; cefotaxime, ceftriaxone, or rarely chloramphenicol if penicillin allergic or suspect ampicillin resistant H. flu or penicillin-resistant pneumococcus (Nejm 1994;331:380), in which case should add vancomycin. In developing countries, alarming appearance of chloro-resistant meningococcus appearing (Nejm 1998;339:868)
- Other gram negatives (Ann IM 1990;112:610): cefotaxime, ceftizoxime, or ceftriaxone for nonpseudomonas types but not Listeria (requires 3 wk penicillin); ceftazidime and gentamicin for Pseudomonas; ampicillin + chloramphenicol or ceftriaxone or cefotaxime for H. flu, and drop the second drug if organism turns out to be ampicillin sensitive
- Unknown adult meningitis: ceftriaxone (1st choice), or cefotaxime (Med Let 1990;32:41) w vancomycin if pneumococcal resistance possible

16.28 NONCHOLERA VIBRIOS: VIBRIO DIARRHEA AND WOUND INFECTIONS

Ann IM 1988;109:261, 318; 1983;99:464; Nejm 1985;312:343
Cause: *Vibrio vulnificus* and *parahaemolyticus*
Epidem: Worldwide (COASTAL) marine seafood, or seawater; causes 1/4 foodborne disease in Japan; various species live in sea, hence GI disease from raw oyster ingestion (Mmwr 1996;45:621), shell cut wound infections, swimming (Ann IM 1983;99:169)
Risk for travelers: Low; but a cause of traveler's diarrhea in raw seafood eaters in Japan, Thailand

Pathophys: Produce enterotoxin and evoke inflammatory mediators

Incubation Period: 12–24 hr

Sx: Nausea, vomiting, diarrhea with cramps, bloody diarrhea in <50%; fever, ha, ear pain; wound pain

Si: Otitis media, cellulitis, gangrene

Crs: 2–4 d (Nejm 1985;312:343)

Cmplc: Septicemia, often fatal, esp in compromised host (Nejm 1979;300:1), such as alcoholics, in whom can cross gut barriers

Lab:

Bact: culture with special medium (TCBS) broth

Rx: Preventive: avoid raw or undercooked seafoods; tetracyclines (Med Let 1991;33:107) or quinolones, but benefit in gastroenteritis questionable

16.29 OTHER STREPTOCOCCAL INFECTIONS: STREPTOCOCCAL ERYSIPELAS, CELLULITIS/WOUND INFECTIONS, NECROTIZING FASCIITIS, AND IMPETIGO

Nejm 1996;334:240

Cause: *Streptococcus pyogenes*, group A, β-hemolytic

Epidem: Worldwide; impetigo more common in tropical areas w poor hygiene (children 2–6); erysipelas and cellulitis, common; necrotizing fasciitis (NF), rare, 1/yr in big hospital; invasive strep infections in 1.5/100,000/yr in general population, 3/1000 of household contacts (Nejm 1996;335:547); but invasive cases are just the tip of the iceberg since same strain will be found causing much more pharyngitis in the community (Jama 1997;277:38)

Risk in travelers: Low = domestic

Incubation period: d to weeks

Pathophys: Erysipelas is mainly in lymphatics; cellulitis, in subcutaneous tissues; NF, infections dissect along fascial planes, so skin is last to go, and look deceptively benign; 1/3 of the time NF is associated with anaerobic bacteria as well; impetigo is a superficial skin infection, starts in a break in the skin

Sx: Pain, fever, and rapid spreading in erysipelas, cellulitis, and NF; in impetigo, sx are of a weeping rash usually in a child

Si: Erysipelas has sharp limits, symmetric swelling, usually across bridge of nose; cellulitis has little edema and indistinct limits; NF has edema, fever, redness, gas crepitation (in 50%), anesthesia (nerve infarction), ecchymosis (thrombosis); in impetigo, rash has bullae with honey yellow exudate

Crs: In NF, 75% die without surgical debridement within 1–2 d

Cmplc: Toxic shock syndrome (16.46) and acute glomerular nephritis can occur with all

Erysipelas: r/o ERYSIPELOID (hands, exposure to raw meat and animals, slower spread; gram-positive rod, culture skin biopsy; rx with penicillin, etc.)

Cellulitis: erythema nodosum and endocarditis, r/o acute axillary lymphadenitis (Nejm 1990;323:655)

NF: r/o gas gangrene

Lab:

Bact: In all, culture, and gram-positive cocci in chains on Gram's stain

Path: for NF, frozen section biopsy

Serol: ASO titers elevated

Rx: Prevention w bacitracin dressing no better than Vaseline (Jama 1996;276:972)

- For all, antibiotics penicillin, erythromycin, although 20–40% resistance now in Finland (Nejm 1992;326:292)
- Impetigo, mupirocin (Bactroban) ointment (not cream) (Rx Let 1998;5:11) topically tid as good as po antibiotics; $10/15-g tube (Med Let 1988;30:55); debated if need to cover for resistant staph, especially nonbullous type (Lancet 1991;338:803)
- NF, extensive surgical debridement first; clindamycin helps decr toxin production

16.30 PARATYPHOID FEVER/SALMONELLOSIS

Cause: *Salmonella paratyphi* and other nontyphoid species

Epidem: Worldwide; incr freq in rainy seasons in tropics; fecal–oral from carriers, 1/3 carry for 1 yr after infection, some forever; birds, esp poultry from GI tracts and including chicken eggs, eg, ice cream epidemic when premix transported in tank truck that had just carried eggs (Nejm 1996;334:1281); beef, especially resistant plasmid-carrying types (Nejm 1987;316:565), epidemics from hamburger, especially in patients on antibiotics; carmine dye (ground-up insects) in food or as stool marker (Nejm 1967;276:829); marijuana (Nejm 1982;306:1249); nosocomial from various sources (Nejm 1968;279:674)

Increased incidence in cancer patients (Nejm 1967;276:1045), 1/400 leukemics, lymphomas, and colon cancer patients; 1/2000 patients with other cancers; 1/9000 patients without cancer

Risk in travelers: Low (2–8% of traveler's diarrhea); incr w gastric achlorhydria, HIV

Pathophys: Endotoxin production by intracellular organisms in small and large bowel

Incubation period: 12–72 hr

Sx: Nausea, vomiting, and diarrhea, sometimes fever

Si: Diarrhea, may be as watery as in cholera

Crs: several day duration; recover spontaneously after 1 wk

Cmplc: Septic arteritis and aneurysms (Nejm 1969;281:310)

Lab:

Bact: Gram-negative rods on stool culture; stool smear with methylene blue shows polys unlike typhoid fever but like other colitis, eg, ulcerative, shigella, *E. coli*, etc. (Ann IM 1972;76:697)

Hem: White counts in normal range, no correlation with severity

Rx: Antibiotics contraindicated for gastroenteritis alone because if rx, then carry in stool longer (27% vs 11% at 31 d), and in vivo resistance develops in 10% (Nejm 1969;281:636); but ciprofloxacin or Tm/S is used if fecal leukocytes, fever, and other measures of severity are bad (Arch IM 1990;150:546); ciprofloxacin does help, but prolongs convalescent excretion (Ann IM 1991;114:195); opiates could theoretically worsen due to decreased motility

Prevent: Standard dietary precautions

16.31 PERTUSSIS (WHOOPING COUGH)

Nejm 1994;331:16

Cause: *Bordetella pertussis* (similar to hemophilus); occasionally sporadically by adenovirus (Nejm 1970;283:390); from respiratory tract of infected persons esp during catarrhal stage; 90% attack rate

Epidem: Worldwide, worst in developing countries; highest incidence in children <5 yr; female morbidity > male; in U.S., increasing to >2500 cases/yr w many infections in adults

Risk for travelers: Incr risk for susceptible travelers to developing countries w low vaccination rates

Pathophys: Rapid bacterial multiplication causes decreased tracheal and bronchial ciliary action which in turn causes infection by strep, staph, etc.; endotoxin produced and released when bacteria die causing cell irritation and occasional death; perhaps neurotoxic effects on CNS; coughing causes anoxia, which somehow causes hemorrhages

Incubation period: 5–20 d

Sx: Catarrhal stage (mild cough) × 2 wk; then paroxysmal coughing; in adults (Ann IM 1998;128:64), nonproductive intermittent chronic cough (>2 wk), 12–21% of those w that sx?! (Jama 1996;275:1672, 1995;273:1044)

Si: Spasmodic coughing, long drawn out with rapid sharp inhalations (whoops); small petechial hemorrhages throughout body

Crs: Paroxysmal stage lasts 2 wk

Cmplc: Seizures; secondary pulmonary infection and atelectasis; meningitis; in infants, apnea and death, 75% are <1 yr, 40% <3 mo (Ann IM 1972;76:289)

Lab:

Bact: culture sputum or nasal/pharyngeal swab during catarrhal stage; smear shows small gram-neg rods, nonmotile, no spores, encapsulated

Hem: WBCs increased with high % (usually >50%) lymphocytes, looks like CLL in a child

Serol: Acutely direct fluorescent antibody (DFA) to the antigen; antibody titer increased after 3 wk

Rx: Preventively (CDC rv-Ann IM 1985;103:896):

• Immunize with antigens 1, 2, and 3 in children between age 6 wk and <6 yr; use acellular pertussis as DTaP for immunizations beginning at 2 mo, 70–90% effective compared to placebo while whole cell vaccine is only 40–60% effective and has encephalitic/neurologic cmplc (Nejm 1996;334:341; 1995;333:1045; Jama 1996;275:37). No cross-placental transfer

• Hyperimmune globulin

- Antibiotics prophylactically or to sick pts to decrease infectivity, do shorten course: erythromycin 40 mg/kg in children, 1 g/d in adults; or Tm/S × 10 d, 8 mg/40 mg/kg in children, 320/1600 in adults

16.32 PLAGUE

Ann Int Med 1995;122:151

Cause: *Yersinia (Pasteurella) pestis*

Epidem: Reports from >15 countries: over $1/2$ E and So Africa, 1/3 Asia, remainder Americas; also Kazakstan, Mongolia

From rats, which eventually die of it, via flea vector; or

- Skin-to-skin contact; or
- Inhalation of respiratory droplets from infected person; or
- Ingestion of respiratory tract excretions

Endemic in western U.S. rodents; found in farm animals too (15 cases/yr in U.S.)

Risk in travelers: Very rare (those at some risk include mammal biologists, others w rodent contact in endemic areas)

Incubation period: 5–7 d

Pathophys: Endotoxin production (Ann IM 1973;79:642), causes DPN inhibition so cell respiration blocked

Sx: Fever, chills, myalgias, ha

Si: Bubo (large node); fever and septicemia; heart block and other conduction abnormalities

Crs: 90% die over 6 d

Cmplc: Pneumonia due to infected thromboemboli or direct infect from others (die in 3 d)

Lab:

Heme: leukocytosis (leukemoid rxn can occur)

Bact: Gram's stain shows gram-negative cocci; culture difficult from blood, nodes; phage diagnosis is specific

Serol: fluorescent antibody

Rx:

- Acute disease, 1st choice, streptomycin; gentamycin can be substituted; also tetracycline, sulfonamides; multidrug resistance reported in Madagascar (Nejm 1997;337:677)

Prevention: Whole cell vaccine (currently not available) is rarely indicated; oral tetracycline have efficacy post-exposure; droplet

precautions until patient is treated 72 hr (pneumonia); standard
precautions for bubonic plague

16.33 PNEUMOCOCCAL INFECTIONS

Cause: *Streptococcus pneumoniae* especially types 3 and 6
(most virulent)

Epidem: Worldwide; population carriers disseminate to pts w
diminished resistance; 50% of population carries in upper
respiratory tract at some time; increased incidence in blood group
A types because pneumococcus has A-like antigens; and in pts
after splenectomy because residual RES requires increased
antibody coating before phagocytosis can occur (Nejm
1981;304:245); marked increased incidence HIV pts; penicillin
resistance rising, already predom in areas of So Africa, Spain, etc.

Risk to travelers: Low = domestic, though may be incr w travel in
temperate densely pop areas such as China

Incubation period: Days to 1 wk

Pathophys: (Nejm 1995;332:1280) Invasive w pyogenic response; little
toxin production; pathogenic via numbers alone; polysaccharide
capsule in virulent strains makes phagocytosis hard

Sx:
    Meningitis: fever, confusion
    Otitis media: ear pain
    Pneumonia: fever, chills, productive cough, sudden onset of pleurisy

Si: Rales
    Meningitis: fever, confusion
    Otitis media: hot ear
    Pneumonia: bloody sputum unlike viral or mycoplasma

Crs:
    Pneumonia: Xray clears in 6 wk (Nejm 1970;283:798)
    Meningitis: 50% mortality

Cmplc: Triad w endocarditis, meningitis, and pneumonia often fatal
(Am J Med 1963;33:262); empyema r/o multiple myeloma if
crit low

Lab:
    Bact: Gram-pos diplococci; culture shows optochin-sensitive/bile salt
soluble colonies

Rx:

- Penicillin iv, though resistance to it and most other β-lactam antibiotics appearing (Nejm 1995;333:481, 1994;331:377, Jama 1994;71:1831); 15% resistance rate to penicillin and ceftazidime and 25% to Tm/S (Jama 1996;275:194), 25% to penicillin nationally (Antimicrob Agents Chemother 1996;40:1208); mortality is not increased when penicillin is used to rx resistant strains (Nejm 1995;333:474)?
- Resistant or possibly resistant pneumococcus: ceftriaxone + vancomycin for life-threatening infections like meningitis; if intermediate resistance, ceftriaxone iv or po levofloxacin or gatifloxacin; if fully resistant, vancomycin iv or po levofloxacin or gatifloxacin, moxafloxacin, etc.

Prevent: 21 strain pneumococcal vaccine, 65% overall effective (Nejm 1991;325:1453; Ann IM 1988;108:653; 1986;104:1–118) at least for elderly and people at increased risk, eg, splenectomy, COPD, alcoholics, diabetes, chronic renal pts on dialysis, CHF (Ann IM 1984;101:325, 348); worth it in all? (Ann IM 1986;104:106 vs Jama 1996;275:194); ineffective in many sick pts who need it the most, eg VA COPD pts (Nejm 1986;315:1318); revaccinate if vaccination in doubt or every 5 yr at least for high risk with new conjugate vaccine effective in children

16.34 PSEUDOMEMBRANOUS COLITIS (*C. DIFFICILE* DIARRHEA)

Nejm 1994;330:257; Med Let 1979;21:97

Cause: *Clostridium difficile*

Epidem: Worldwide; associated with antibiotic rx, usually broad-spectrum types and especially clindamycin; also the cause of 20% of all antibiotic-associated diarrhea without pseudomembranous colitis

Risk for travelers: Always a consideration in travelers w persistent diarrhea after antibiotic treatment

Pathophys: Proliferates when there is suppression of normal bowel flora by various broad-spectrum antibiotics; cytotoxic toxin production

Incubation period: days to 6 wk

Sx: H/o antibiotic use, esp cephalosporin or clindamycin >6 d before loose but not watery diarrhea onset; occasionally fever, abdominal pain

Si: Raised plaques (pseudopolyps) on sigmoidoscopy or colonoscopy, "swollen rice grains," bleed when scraped; rectum may be spared often

Crs: Often self-limited w stop of antibiotics

Cmplc: 15–20% relapse rate w rx, rare toxic megacolon

Lab:

   Bact: fecal leukocytes by methylene blue stain or Gram's stain of stool

   Chem: Toxin assayable in stool by various methods; by tissue culture assay, 94–100% sens, 99% specif; by latex agglutination assay (poorest test but most often used), 50% sens, 99% specif; by enzyme-linked methods, 75% sens, 99% specif; order if positive fecal leukocytes stain

   Hem: Increased polys

Rx: (Med Let 1989;31:94); colitis; stop antibiotics and give metronidazole (Flagyl) 250 mg po qid × 10–14 d, perhaps iv if ileus; as good as vancomycin and costs a small fraction of what vanco costs (Lancet 1983;2:1043); or vancomycin 125 mg po qid × 10–14 d, increase to 500 mg qid in resistant cases but do not give iv since is not secreted into bowel where the organism is

Prevent: Cautious use clindamycin and other anbiotic use (Ann IM 1994;120:272)

16.35 PSITTACOSIS

Nejm 1986;315:189

Cause: *Chlamydia psittaci*

Epidem: North America, Central America, Europe; birds such as parakeets, parrots, chickens, pigeons; fecal spread; 100–200 cases from birds/yr in U.S.; assoc w caged parrot ownership in tropics

Risk for travelers: Rare = domestic U.S. risk

Pathophys: Intracellular infx w secondary inflammatory response

Incubation period: 7–14 d

Si: Prominent headache; fever; sore throat, dry cough confusion, headache, and muscle spasms mimic meningitis; pneumonitis;

bradycardia relative to temperature; r/o gm-neg shock, typhoid
(16.51), yellow fever, Q fever (16.36)

Crs: 10–21 d, 20% fatal without rx

Cmplc: R/o mycoplasma (cold agglutinins), Q fever (antibody titers),
strep, and staph

Lab:

Bact: culture blood, sputum

Hem: ESR low frequently, r/o trichinosis, leptospirosis (16.22),
brucellosis (16.8), legionnaire's (16.20), Q fever (16.36), other
pneumonias

Serol: Complement-fixing antibody on paired sera, r/o
lymphogranuloma venereum

Rx: Tetracycline or erythromycin 500 mg qid × 2–3 wk

Prevent: Avoid bird contact unless declared disease free by vet, pet store,
owner, etc.

16.36 Q FEVER

Nejm 1988;319:354; CID 1995;20:489; Am J Med 1992;93:427

Cause: *Coxiella burnetii*

Epidem: Worldwide; airborne, eg, in hay; animal reservoirs (stock
animals, and cats, especially parturient ones); tick vector from
mouse reservoir; milk from chronically infected cows; resists
dessication

Risk for travelers: Low = U.S. domestic but higher in sheep raising areas
France, So Europe, Australia

Pathophys: Intracellular in vessel endothelium

Incubation period: 14–39 d (average 20 d); mos for endocarditis

Sx: Fever, headache, pains in muscles and chest wall; sudden onset;
sometimes nonproductive cough; rare rash

Si:

Cardiovascular: relative bradycardia, migratory thrombophlebitis

Skin: papule, then vesicle and eschar after 3–4 wk (rare)

Pulmonary: patchy pneumonitis, dry cough, pleurisy

GI: hepatitis (Ann IM 1971;74:198); hepatosplenomegaly (50%)

Rheumatoid: migratory arthritis

Crs: 2–4 wk; 10–90 d for pneumonia

Cmplc: Endocarditis (rare); meningoencephalitis; pericarditis/myocarditis

Lab:
    Heme: Normal WBC (90%); decr plts (25%)
    Chem: Incr LFTs (85%)
    Bact: Culture not routinely possible: fastidious grower, needs high CO_2, low O_2
    Serol: Seroconversion 7–15 d; ELISA, microimmunofluorescence; IFA current reference test; antibody elevated; phase 2 > phase 1 in acute disease; phase 1 incr in chronic disease; use same antigens used to test for typhus, Weil–Felix negative (r/o rickettsial pox); test confounded by presence of rheumatoid factor; overall sens >80% after 1 wk; specificity 90%

Rx: Tetracycline (usually doxycycline 200 mg/d × 14–21 d); quinolones may have activity; macrolides questionable

Prevent: Avoid close contact (aerosols) w animals that are giving birth; whole cell vaccine available in Australia only

16.37 RAT BITE FEVER

Am J Med 1988;85:711; Lancet 1987;2:1361; Ann IM 1969;71:979

Cause: *Streptobacillus moniliformis,* occasionally *Spirillum minus* (a spirochete)

Epidem: Worldwide; rat bite or contaminated dairy products (Haverhill fever); in low socioeconomic groups and in medical researchers working with rats

Risk to travelers: Very rare = domestic

Incubation period: 1–22 d

Pathophys: Usual innoc w bite, then bacteremia w tissue invasion

Sx: Bitten 2–3 d before, heals in 10–12 d; very inflamed bite in case of *Spirillum;* both cause fever, chills; arthralgias in large joints, rash

Si: Fever, macular or petechial rash on palms and soles; w spirillosis, ulceration at bite

Crs: Relapsing fever w rash may occur w spirillosis for wks, shorter course for *Streptobacillus*

Cmplc: Endocarditis and other cardiac infections; r/o rickettsia, Coxsackie B, Lyme, relapsing fever, pasteurellosis, syphilis, gonococcal infx

Lab: Note that false pos RPR may occur w either infx

Bact: blood culture positive for *Streptobacillus*; spirillum can be seen on peripheral smear w darkfield

Rx: Use gloves preventively; penicillin for all types (Ann IM 1985;102:229)

Prevent: Pasteurized dairy products; limit contact w rodent infested areas

16.38 RELAPSING FEVER

Nejm 1993;329:939

Cause: *Borrelia recurrentis*, B. hermsii, others

Epidem: Worldwide, but especially w foci in U.S., Central and So America, Africa, Asia; see Fig. 16.1, epidemic form via louse vector carrying person to person; endemic form via soft (argasid) tick vector carrying between animal reservoirs to humans; outbreaks in U.S. in campers using mountain cabins

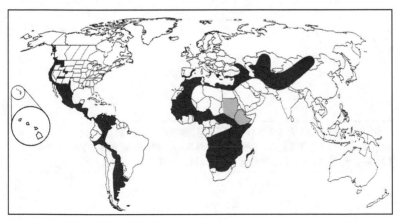

Relapsing Fever
☐ Louse-borne relapsing fever
■ Tick-borne relapsing fever

Figure 16.1. Distribution of relapsing fever. (Reproduced with permission from *Tropical Infectious Diseases*.)

Risk for travelers: Rare; exposure to tick-borne disease in rustic cabins in western U.S.; louse-borne disease requires local contact in refugee or other disrupted environment where epidemic disease established

Pathophys: Organism changes antigen structure q 1–2 wk and causes bacteremia, which causes antibody production leading to antigen–antibody rosettes, which cause vasculitis and then sx subside again

Incubation period: 5–10 d

Sx: Headache, fever, chills, myalgias, arthralgias, abdominal pain

Si: Each attack is 3–5 d of fever, then 4–10 d afebrile; rash may be macular, papular, or purpuric looking like meningococcal bacteremia; hepatosplenomegaly

Crs: 3–10 recurrent attacks unless rx

Cmplc: Meningoencephalitis, cranial neuritis; epidemic type has up to 50% mortality; endemic form has <2% mortality

Lab:

Bact: Buffy coat smear shows spirochetes, loosely coiled by darkfield, or Giemsa or Wright's stain; rat inoculation shows positive buffy coat changes as above in 4 d

Hem: elevated wbc and ESR; low platelets

Rx: 1st, tetracycline or doxycycline (100 mg bid for 10 d); 2nd, streptomycin; 3rd, penicillin, which commonly causes Herxheimer's reaction (J Inf Dis 1978;137:573), like syphilis (16.44)

Prevent: Insecticide use in cabins or dwellings w rodents (and their soft ticks) may decr risk for tick-borne disease

---

16.39 ROCKY MOUNTAIN SPOTTED FEVER AND OTHER SPOTTED FEVER GROUP RICKETTSIAS (RMSF, TICK TYPHUS, BOUTONNEUSE FEVER)

Nejm 1993;329:941; Ann IM 1976;84:752

Cause: *Rickettsia rickettsii* (Western hemishpere), *R. conorii* (Mediterranean), *R. australis* (Australia), *R. japonica* (Asia), *R. africae* (Africa, Guadeloupe; Nejm 2001;344:1504)

Epidem: No and So America, Mediterranean, So Europe, Middle East, E Africa, So Africa, eastern Australia; carried by ticks (large and visible) from wild rodent reservoirs; *Dermacentor* ticks in No

America, *Amblyomma* and *Rhipicephalus* in So America; endemic in Rocky Mountain rodents; also on Cape Cod and throughout most mid-Atlantic states including Virginia and North Carolina; also seen in lab technicians working with ticks; 700–1000 cases/yr in U.S.; see Fig. 16.2

Risk for travelers: Imported cases in U.S. are mainly in safari participants, adventure travelers, military (African tick typhus); U.S. risk highest in southeastern Atlantic states, esp No Carolina; occurred in 14% of U.S. troops in Botswana (Emerging Inf Dis 1996;2:217)

Pathophys: Angiitis due to endothelial infection causing proliferation and thrombosis via activation of kallikrein–kinin system (Ann IM 1978;88:764); subclinical DIC changes in platelet and clotting system detectable even before sx (Nejm 1988;318:1021)

Incubation period: 5–7 d

Sx: Seasonal; 95% of cases between April and August; tick bite (most recall) or dog contact; incubation period, 5–7 d; severe frontal headache (90%) is usually first sx; myalgias (80%), emesis (60%)

Si: Rash (90% after 4–5 d), centripetal progression (extremities to trunk), palm and sole involved (in 2/12); toxic with fever leading to confusion (in 10/13); muscle tenderness, especially calf and thigh; diffuse angiitis; skin necrosis regardless of pressure points; African tick typhus and Mediterranean boutonneuse fever cause eschar at bite w dark crust; may be multiple

Cmplc: Mortality without rx = 25%; w rx, 5%; carditis, cerebral edema, DIC

- r/o babesiosis; rat bite fever (16.37); RICKETTSIAL POX (Nejm 1994;331:1612) from *Rickettsia akari*, seen all over U.S., initial lesion at mouse mite bite, 1 wk latency then fever, malaise, and chicken pox-like vesicular lesions, not too sick, can rx w tetracycline

Lab:

Hem: thrombocytopenia (Nejm 1969;280:58) and DIC

Path: skin bx of rash positive on immunofluorescent stain (available from CDC)

Serol: antibody increased by immunofluorescence or microagglutination by day 15; western blot for confirmation of rickettsial type; PCR also effective (Nejm 2001;344:1504); in Rocky Mountain spotted fever, OX2 and OX19 positive, OXK negative; in rickettsial pox, all neg

Rickettsiae of the Spotted Fever Group

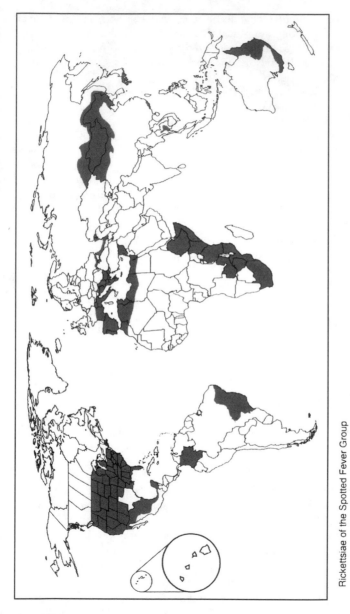

Figure 16.2. Distribution of rickettsias of the spotted fever group. (Reproduced with permission from Tropical Infectious Diseases.)

Rx: 1st, tetracycline; or 2nd, chloramphenicol, usual Rx 7 d, but for African tick typhus and Mediterranean tick fever, 1 d may be sufficient (Nejm 2001;344:1504)

Prevent: DEET-containing repellants, permethrin treated clothing (see 16.37)

16.40 SCARLET FEVER/ STREPTOCOCCAL TOXIC SHOCK

Nejm 1970;282:23; 1970;297:365

Cause: Toxin producing strains of *Streptococcus pyogenes* (rarely *Staph. aureus*, which causes no sore throat)

Epidem: Worldwide; respiratory droplets and wound infections; occurs in children only, since adults usually already immune

Risk to travelers: Rare = domestic

Incubation period: days to 1 wk

Pathophys: Erythrogenic toxin produced by bacteria lysogenized by a specific phage which causes bacterial capsular dilatation, rupture, and toxin release

Sx: Sore throat, fever, rash; w TSS, nausea, vomiting, soft tissue swelling, dizziness

Si: Rash, trunkal, especially in creases (Pastia's lines) palpable, viral-like; spots on soft palate; "strawberry" tongue; circumoral pallor; w TSS, hypotension, often cellulitis/fasciitis, erythroderm, etc.

Crs: Variable, self-limited (pharyngitis) to fatal (streptococcal toxic shock, necrotizing fasciitis, etc.)

Cmplc:
- Acute glomerular nephritis
- Rheumatic fever, in old days 3% in epidemic and 1/2% in endemic type if no rx; now <1/10,000 without rx, and <1/100,000 with rx in adults
- Peritonsillar abscess (Quincy abscess), and tonsillar vein phlebitis leading to pulmonary emboli, rx with tonsillectomy
- Toxic shock syndrome, which may just be the extreme variant (Nejm 1991;325:783)
- R/o other childhood exanthems: roseola, rubeola, rubella, ehrlichia (16.17); in tropics must consider other entities as in staph TSS (16.46), leptospirosis (16.22), rickettsial (16.39, 16.57)

Lab: Sore throat workup protocol (Ann IM 1980;93:244)

    Bact: throat culture, single swab positive in 75%, 2 swabs in 85%
β-hemolysis on culture plates; positive culture may still be just a
carrier; rapid office tests take 10 min–1 hr, cost $2–$3 plus lots
of time (Med Let 1985;27:49) but may still have to culture if
negative (J Ped 1987;111:80)

    Hem: eosinophils increased often

Rx: Penicillin, erythromycin; if sick, treatment speeds healing
(Jama 1975;227:1278); but overall often does not (Am J Med
1951;10:300); for toxic shock, IV clindamycin plus penicillin
+/– IV immune globulin and surgery to necrotic tissue areas

Prevent: None

16.41 SCRUB TYPHUS

Cause: *Orientia tsutsugamushi*

Epidem: Rural and suburban So Asia, W Pacific (Malaysia, Indonesia,
Papua New Guinea); transmitted by larval mites (chiggers);
accounts for 20% admits for fever in peninsular Malaysia

Risk for travelers: Low, but incr risk in recent yrs reported

Incubation period: 6–20 d

Sx: Fever, headache, loss of hearing (1/3)

Si: Eschar at site of bite (1/3–1/2), lymphadenopathy, conjunctival
suffusion, transient truncal rash

Crs: Mild to fatal

Cmplc: Rare seizure, coma

Lab: Leukopenia, thrombocytopenia

    Serol: IFA, dot blot enzyme immunoassay

Rx: Doxykycline (100 mg bid) plus rifampin (Lancet 2000;356:1057);
report of doxycyline resistance from No Thailand

Prevent: Doxycycline 200 mg/wk is protective (JID 1982;146:811)

16.42 STAPH FOOD POISONING

Nejm 1984;310:1368, 1437
Cause: *Staphylococcus aureus*
Epidem: Worldwide—esp hot climates; most common type of food poisoning
Risk to travelers: Similar to domestic risk, but may be incr in hot climates w inadequate use of refrigeration
Incubation period: 2–6 hr
Pathophys: Heat-stable enterotoxin produced by staph in food after preparation, eg, potato salad; lack of fever indicates a toxin disease
Sx: Nausea, vomiting, and some diarrhea without fever; excess nausea and vomiting relative to diarrhea suggests staph rather than others
Crs: Resolves in 24–72 hr
Cmplc: R/o clostridial and *Bacillus cereus* food poisonings, both of which also lack fever
Lab: None unless need to work up for public health reasons, then Gram's stain and culture the food
Rx: Symptomatic
Prevent: Avoid perishable foods (dairy products, creamy desserts, etc.) served at room temperature

16.43 STAPHYLOCOCCAL SOFT TISSUE INFECTIONS (FURUNCULOSIS, CELLULITIS, PYOMYOSITIS)

Nejm 1998;338:520
Cause: *Staphylococcus aureus*
Epidem: Worldwide; pyomyositis (muscle abcess) much commoner in tropics; normal inhabitant of skin and upper respiratory track; 90% resistant to penicillin
Risk to travelers: Similar to nontraveler, though furuncular disease more common in hot humid climates; pyomyositis much more common in tropics than temperate regions
Incubation period: Variable

Pathophys: Multiple exotoxins increase its pathogenicity including β-lactamase, coagulase, hyaluronidase, other proteases, leukocidin, lipases, hair follicles infected because fibrin restrains spread but retards healing; mech for development of infx of large muscles w pyomyositis unknown

Sx: Cellulitis: pain, swelling, may have fever; furunculosis: painful boils; pyomyositis: fever, swelling and pain over large muscle group that may persist for wks

Si: Abscesses, carbuncle, furuncle, pyomyositis causes woody induration over affected muscle

Crs: Pyomyositis mort 1%, but responds well to drainage

Cmplc: Bacteremia: DIC, endocarditis including R-sided especially in drug users, metastatic infections

Lab:

Bact: Gram-positive cocci clusters, coagulase-positive; methicillin resistance present in over 50% in ICUs (Nejm 1998;339:520)

Rx: Surgical drainage of pyomyositis, furuncles, other abcess
- β-Lactamase-resistant drug such as nafcillin/oxacillin iv, later go to po cloxacillin or diclox; cephalosporin, clindamycin, Tm/S, erythromycin
- Methicillin-resistant staph (Nejm 1989;320:1188): 1st, vancomycin (Med Let 1982;24:107) w or without rifampin for endocarditis, although time to bacteremic clearing in SBE may be up to 2 wk (Ann IM 1991;115:674); or 2nd, Tm/S (Ann IM 1992;117:390), minocycline, fluoroquinolones, clindamycin

Prevent: Recurrent abscesses: prevent w rifampin 600 mg bid × 5 d (Nejm 1986;315:91) + clindamycin, flouroquinolone, or Tm/S (Ann IM 1982;97:317); topical antibiotics, especially mupirocin to the anterior nares to eliminate carrier states especially of methicillin-resistant staph (Ann IM 1991;14:101)

16.44 SYPHILIS

Nejm 1992;326:1060

Cause: *Treponema pallidum*

Epidem: Worldwide; incidence = 20+/100,000 in U.S., increasing since 1985; spread via direct contact (venereal) with primary (1°) or secondary (2°) lesion

Risk for travelers: Low, assoc w unprotected sexual contact

Pathophys: In 2°, marked bacteremia is present; tertiary (3°) types probably represent hypersensitivity reactions since few organisms are present; gummas, from endarteritis obliterans which causes necrosis, eg, in aortic media. Three types of neurosyphilis:

- TABES DORSALIS
- Meningovascular
- General paresis

All 3° complications are increased in AIDS (Nejm 1987;316:1600)

Sx:

1°: painless chancre

2°: rash, round with pigmented center; fever; headache; alopecia; eye pain from iritis

Si:

1°: chancre with edema (looks like squamous cell cancer), and nonsuppurative lymphadenitis

2°: macular/papular/pustular rash with pustules, annular-appearing as ages, on palms and soles; split papules at mouth corners and other moist body areas (condyloma lata); diffuse lymphadenopathy; meningitis

3°:

- Neurosyphilis: Argyle-Robertson pupils (small, unequal, reactive to accommodation not light); general paresis dementia; meningovascular, strokes, meningitis and cranial nerve palsies (Nejm 1994;331:1469, 1516) most commonly seen within 3–4 yr of primary infection especially in AIDS pts, tabes dorsalis with motor long tract and sensory losses usually in lower extremities
- Vascular including aortitis with AI and aneurysms in 10%
- Gummas in 15%; 75% are cutaneous

Congenital: onset at age 14+ weeks even if seronegative at birth; si: rash, fever, hepatosplenomegaly, rhinitis, lymphadenopathy, elevated LFTs, CSF cells, and protein (Nejm 1990;323:1299); notched permanent (Hutchinson's) teeth, in 25%; interstitial keratitis in 50%; saddle nose

Crs: 1°: 9–90 d, 20–30% develop secondary syphilis; 2°: months if no rx

Cmplc: 1°: r/o herpes and chancroid (both tender); 2°: obstructive pattern hepatitis (Nejm 1971;284:1422); nephrosis from immune complex disease (Nejm 1975;292:449); 3°: cirrhosis (Med Clin N Am 1964;48:613)

R/o BEJEL and PINTA from *Treponema carateum*, spread by skin-to-skin contact with lesions, as well as by flies in pinta; bejel in Arabia, pinta in Central and South America; primary disease consists of a nonulcerating papule; secondary, of pigmented skin lesions later becoming depigmented and hyperkeratotic; tertiary of cardiovascular and nervous system involvement; rx w penicillin

R/o YAWS from *T. pertenue*, spread skin-to-skin in many tropical areas, especially affecting children; an ulcerating papule w "strawberry" scar formation; rx w penicillin

Lab:

Bact: Darkfield shows bacteria with 8–14 spirals, ~7 m long; false positives in mouth from normal treponema flora there

CSF: do LP 1 yr post rx of 1° or 2° types if VDRL or FTA still positive; in meningovascular syphilis elevated protein, and cells are present; VDRL positive in 50% but can be negative even if bacteria present, getting FTA hence better; probably best to just rx for 3–4 wk without LP if asx (Ann IM 1986;104:86)

Serol: (review; Ann IM 1986;104:368)

- VDRL or RPR is positive in 76% of 1° cases (if negative, darkfield positive still), 100% of 2° cases; and 75% of 3° cases; false pos (>1/16) in mononucleosis, malaria, collagen vascular diseases, sarcoid, leprosy, yaws, pinta
- TPI is positive in 50% of 1°, 98% of 2°, and 90% of 3° cases
- FTA (Nejm 1969;280:1086) positive in 90% primaries, 99% secondaries, 98% tertiaries; false positives in only 30% VDRL false-positive patients, some with yaws, pinta, or in 10% lupus but is atypical (beaded; Nejm 1970;282:1287); remains positive all life

Xray: Congenital type has lytic areas (bites) in long bones, subperiosteal

Rx: (Med Let 1994;36:1) same even if HIV positive (Nejm 1997;337:307); prevent by partner notification, usefulness limited (Ann IM 1990;112:539)

- Early disease (1°, 2°, or latent <1 yr): 1st, benzathine penicillin (Bicillin) 2.4 million U im × 1; or 2nd, doxycycline 100 mg po bid × 14 d; or 3rd, erythromycin 500 mg po qid × 14 d
- Late, short of neurosyphilis: 1st, benzathine penicillin 2.4 million U im weekly × 3 wk; or 2nd, doxycycline 100 mg po bid × 4 wk
- Neurosyphilis: penicillin G 2–4 million U iv q 4 h × 10–14 d, or procaine penicillin 2.4 million U im + probenecid (Benemid) 500 mg po qid × 10–14 d

- Congenital: penicillin G 50,000 U/kg im/iv q 8–12 h × 10–14 d, or procaine penicillin 50,000 U/kg im qd × 10–14 d
- If penicillin allergy: ceftriaxone im qd × 10 d, or tetracycline 2 g qd or doxycycline 100 mg po bid × 15 d (12% failure rate) or erythromycin 2 g qd × 10 d (30 d for tertiary) (12% failure rate); rx for 28 d if late latent disease <1% relapse; follow VDRL, goes negative in 3–6 mo; with CNS lues, follow CSF cells; Herxheimer's reaction (endotoxin sx with fever) within hours after penicillin (Nejm 1976;295:21); longer rx in AIDS where early neurosyphilis develops (Nejm 1994;331:1469; Ann IM 1991;114:872; 1988;109:855) and penicillin rx only transiently effective since long-term cure normally depends on immunity

16.45 TETANUS AND LOCKJAW

Nejm 1973;289:1293; 1969;280:569

Cause: *Clostridium tetani*, via wound contamination with dirt

Epidem: Worldwide; one million cases annually; common in developing countries; present in most soils; 535 cases in 1965 in U.S.; ~4 cases/100 million, mainly in southern states; Texas had 56% of cases; highest incidence in very young and very old (inadequate immunization); <3% of patients have hx of ever having had tetanus toxoid; increased incidence in "skin popping" drug addicts; females > males

Risk for travelers: None, if tetanus boosters are up to date; but puncture wounds not uncommon in travelers, partic w ecotourism, etc., so immunization status important

Pathophys: Exotoxin production and transported both via circulation to CNS (probably most significant in humans), and along motor nerves to CNS (but cannot correlate wound distance from CNS with morbidity and mortality in humans)

Incubation period: 1–54 d (median 8 d)

Sx: Puncture wound or laceration (58%), or postpartum, postsurgery, skin ulcers

Si: Spastic paralysis; tonic convulsive contractions precipitated by intrinsic or extrinsic muscle movement; no or rarely fever

Crs: 60% mortality

Cmplc: R/o "STIFF MAN SYNDROME," autoimmune antibodies against GABA neurons (Nejm 1990;322:1555) induced muscle spasms over years, seen with hypopituitarism, IDDM, Graves', and other endocrinopathies (Nejm 1988;318:1012; 1984;310:1511); occasionally is an autoimmune paraneoplastic syndrome in breast cancer (Nejm 1993;328:546); r/o malignant neuroleptic syndrome

Lab:

Bact: smears show gram-pos bacilli; culture shows fastidious anaerobe, pos in 32% of proven cases

Rx: Prevent w toxoid vaccine (CDC review; Ann IM 1985;103:896) im, primary series of 3 over 1 yr, then q 10 yr, more frequently increases risk of reaction without increasing protection (Nejm 1969;280:575); some argue that routine dT booster is unnecessary in adults (Lancet 5/11/85, p1089); booster of dT is enough even for dirty wounds if last dT was less than 5 yr ago (Nejm 1983;309:636)

Tetanus human immune globulin 250 U im, for dirty wounds with vaccine if not sure has had primary series; give coincident with vaccine in different im area; of disease: metronidazole 500 mg iv q 6 h (Nejm 1995;332:812); human immune globulin; respirator (Ann IM 1978;88:66)

16.46 TOXIC SHOCK SYNDROME (STAPHYLOCOCCAL): DDX IN TROPICAL TRAVELER

Nejm 1998;339:527; Ann IM 1982;96(2)-whole issue is review; 1982;97:608

Cause: *Staph. aureus;* occasionally strep-induced (Nejm 1987;317:146) by group A *Strep. pyogenes,* which produces scarlet fever toxin A (Nejm 1991;325:783; 1989;321:1)

Epidem: Initially 97% cases were associated with tampon use during menses, now none is w change in tampon manufacture, but 2/3 of cases still assoc w menstuation; associated w influenza (Jama 1987;257:1053); nonmenstrual cases assoc w skin lesions, wounds, postpartum, etc.

Risk to travelers: Similar to U.S. risk (low); presentation may be mimicked by several tropical diseases (see below)

Pathophys: Enterotoxins (TSST-1 and others) produced at any body site

Sx: Diarrhea (98%), vomiting (92%), headache, dizziness, sore throat (77%), myalgias, rash

Si: Fever (87%), hypotension, scarlatiniform or macular rash, which later desquamates; conjuctival injection; strawberry tongue

Crs: 10–15% mortality

Cmplc: Hepatitis and renal failure; recurrent (up to 25%), but less severe w recurrences; chronic headache and memory changes (Ann IM 1982;96:865); r/o rickettsial (16.39, 16.57); leptospirosis (16.22); dengue (20.5, 20.17); viral hemorrhagic fevers (20.3, 20.4, 20.6, 20.13), ehrlichiosis (16.17), Kawasaki' s disease

Lab:
  Bact: *Staph. aureus* (TSST-1 producing) in cultures of infected site, blood cultures usually negative

Rx: Fluids, staph antibiotics like clindamycin, which shut down toxin production; perhaps steroids, perhaps immune globulin; remove any foreign or drainable source

16.47 TRAVELER'S DIARRHEA (ESP TOXIGENIC E. COLI)

Nejm 1993;328:1821; Lancet 2000;356:133.

Cause: *E. coli*, esp enterotoxigenic; less commonly enteroadherent, rarely enterohemorrhagic; also sometimes *Campylobacter* (esp in winter), *Shigella*, *Salmonella*, *Vibrios* (coastal SE Asia), *Giardia*, *Cyclospora*, viral, etc.

Epidem: Worldwide, but partic assoc w travel from developed areas to developing areas of tropics/subtropics; in salads and other perishable foods, sewer-contaminated water; 30% of all travelers to Mexico get one type or the other, usually within 2 wk of arrival (Nejm 1976;294:1299); similar rates to other areas, though may be lower in winter; highest incidence in first 2 wks, but can occur anytime (Jama 1999;281:811); toxin types represent 75% of all traveler's diarrhea

Risk to travelers: Moderate to high for travel to developing countries (5–60%); over 7 million cases/yr in travelers (CID 2000;31:1079)

Pathophys: For enterotoxigenic *E. coli*—a toxin is produced while the organisms are attached to gut wall much like *C. perfringens*;

heat-labile toxin type is delayed in onset like cholera; heat-stable types cause immediate onset (Nejm 1975;292:933); in the unusual invasive types, colonic wall invasion causes bloody mucus, like *Shigella*

Sx: Toxin-producing types: clear, watery diarrhea, abdominal cramps; uncommonly fever

Si: Toxin-producing types: sometimes low-grade fever; in invasive types, fever

Crs: Average duration 3–7 d; fewer than 5% persist for >30 d

Cmplc: R/o other GI infections

Lab: For persistent diarrhea or severe sx: obtain stool culture, stool for O + P and/or stool *Giardia* antigen; also consider stool for detection of *C. difficile* toxin if hx of antibiotic use

Rx: Diarrheal sx when traveling with loperamide + antibiotic (Ann Int Med 1991;114:731); shorten course from 80 hr to 24 hr; 80% of travelers report effectiveness (Am J Trop Med Hyg 2000;62:585)

- Ciprofloxacin, 1st choice, 500 mg po bid × 1–3 d (Ann IM 1991;114:731), also gets most *Campylobacter*, *Salmonella*, and *Shigella* as well as the pathogenic *E. coli*; or norfloxacin 400 mg po bid × 1–3 d; or ofloxacin (Floxin) 300 mg po bid × 1–3 d; or levofloxacin 500 mg/d; single dose may be effective (Lancet 1994;344:1537)
- Azithromycin (500 mg/d × 1, then 250 mg/d × 1–2 d; pediatric dose 10 mg/kg/d × 1, then 5 mg/kg/d × 1–2)
- Loperamide HCl (Imodium) 4 mg po then 2 mg after each stool up to 16 mg po qd used with any antibiotic below does not hurt, may help (Ann IM 1993;118:377; 1991;114:731); diphenoxylate + atropine (Lomotil) may worsen some types, eg, *Shigella* (Jama 1973;226:1575); may be benefit of antisecretory drugs (ie, provir); see also antimicrobial agents (Chemother 2001;45:212)

Prevent: Food water precautions; in travelers willing to risk antibiotic rx cmplc's (which, rarely, can even be fatal) rx of sx may be the better approach): see Chapter 5

- Ciprofloxacin, 1st choice, 500 mg po (Lancet 1994;334:1537) qd; or ofloxacin (Floxin) 300 mg po qd; or norfloxacin 400 mg po qd
- Doxycycline 100 mg qd × 5 wk (90% effective, Nejm 1978;298:758) but resistance common in 1993; GI excretion means can use in face of renal or hepatic disease

- Pepto-Bismol 60 cc or ii tabs qid (75% effective), has 2 ASA equivalents/60 cc (Med Let 1980;22:63); salicylate probably inhibits prostaglandins, hence effect or antibiotic effect of bismuth
- Tm/S SS po qd in children, risks allergic reaction

16.48 TRENCH FEVER

Ann IM 1973;79:26
Cause: *Bartonella quintana*
Epidem: Worldwide; body louse, person to person; alcoholic, homeless, and AIDS pts (Nejm 1995;332:419, 424); Europe, USSR, Mexico
Risk for travelers: Rare—assoc w poor living conditions
Incubation period: 3–38 d
Pathophys: Inflammatory/neovascular visceral lesions
Sx: Fever, headache, myalgias
Si: Conjunctival injection, rash, hepatosplenomegaly
Crs: Relapsing or continuous fever for 2–6 wk (each episode lasting 4–6 d)
Cmplc: Endocarditis; and bacillary angiomatosis (Nejm 1997;337:1876; 1995;332:419) cutaneous and deep tissue infections as well as osteolytic bone lesions, esp in AIDS and other immunocompromised pts
Lab:
  Bact: small pleomorphic gram-neg
  Serol: comp-fix antibody; Weil–Felix OXK positive ST, 50% never become OXK Weil–Felix positive; fluorescent antibody increased × 4 in 100%
Rx: Macrolide antibiotics, tetracyclines, chloramphenicol
Prevent: Delousing treatments; improved hygiene, living conditions

16.49 TUBERCULOSIS

Am J Respir Crit Care Med 1994;149:1359; Ann IM 1993;119:400;
  Nejm 1998;338:1641

Cause: *Mycobacterium tuberculosis* and *bovis*

Epidem: Worldwide; recent incr in eastern Europe; drug resistance an
  incr problem in countries w/o infrastructure for rx; spread by
  Inhalation of respiratory droplets of infected persons; but once on
  drugs probably little infectivity despite positive smears (Nejm
  1974;290:459); reinfection may be as important as reactivation, at
  least in homeless; incidence, 25,000 new U.S. cases/yr; these rates
  are increased in the 1990s from HIV patients, prisons, homeless
  populations (Nejm 1992;326:703), and the foreign born (Jama
  1997;278:304); 40% of U.S. cases now occur in foreign born
  (Jama 2000;284:2894), 3/4 cases from patients with previous
  positive PPD, 25 million positive PPDs in U.S., only 5–10% ever
  result in active disease whereas HIV pos pts who contract tbc
  become active cases at 5–10%/yr; in elderly and foreign born,
  90% of cases are reactivation, whereas only 60% are in younger
  pts and the homeless (Jama 1996;275:305), and 1/3 are recent
  infections (Nejm 1994;330:1692)

Incidence higher in diabetics, institutionalized, household contacts,
  HIV-infected (Nejm 1992;326:231; 1991;324:289), alcoholics,
  gastrectomy, silicosis, immunosuppressed, postpartum (Ann IM
  1971;74:764) patients, blacks (Ncjm 1990;322:422), and w highly
  virulent strains (Nejm 1998;338:633)

M. bovis now very rare in developed countries due to pasteurization
  of milk

Worldwide 33% prevalence and causes 6% of all deaths
  (Jama 1995;273:220; Mmwr1993;42:961)

Risk to travelers: Low, but incr in some urban areas; long-term
  travelers/workers to areas of high endemicity run substantial risk
  (3.5 cases/1000 person-mos; Lancet 2000;356:461); risks incr 3×
  for health care workers; risk of exposure to multidrug res strains
  greatest in former USSR, Asia, Dominican Republic, Argentina
  (Nejm 1998;338:1641)

Pathophys: (Nejm 1967;277:1008)
  • Primary infection by inhalation to lower lungs leading to local node
    involvement and asx bacteremia causing gradual hypersensitization

via lymphocytic response and eventual calcification and scar = sterile Ghon complex

- Secondary disease is a reactivation and hypersensitivity reaction to bacteria spread by asx bacteremia to lung apices and upper kidneys where high O_2 concentrations prevent Ghon complex-type sterilization

Sx: Fever, weight loss, night sweats, cough, sputum production, hemoptysis

Si: Same as sx

Crs: Mortality 6%/yr, 12% at 2 yr but 50% at 2 yr if HIV pos and 80% if have AIDS (Jama 1996;276:1223)

Cmplc:

- Apical lung abscess; peritonitis (Nejm 1969;281:1091); meningitis; epididymitis; PID; endometritis; splenic and hepatic abscesses; nontender, scarring skin sores/abscesses; arthritis (especially *M. bovis*); pericarditis (Nejm 1964;270:327); osteomyelitis, especially of spine (POTT'S DISEASE); pleuritis (Am Rev Tbc 1955;71:616); laryngitis, very infectious (Ann IM 1974;80:708); hypercalcemia (25%) from vitamin D sensitivity (Ann IM 1979;90:324)
- Antibiotic resistance, geographically variable, 25% of cases resistant to INH and/or rifampin (Nejm 1993;328:521; 1998;338:1641); multiple drug resistance epidemics in AIDS patients now (Nejm 1992;326:1514) esp in New York City (Jama 1996;276:1229)

Lab:

Bact: sputum or urine AFB smears; tuberculostearic acid assay better than smear (Ann IM 1989;111:650); cultures of sputum, gastric aspirate, urine, peritoneal fluid (1 L spun down; Nejm 1969;281:1091); RIAs now possible in 3 wk

Path: biopsy of liver pos in high % of miliary, or of peritoneum if ascites protein >2.5 gm % (64% true pos; Nejm 1969;281:1091)

Skin tests: intermediate strength (IPPD, 5 U), positive if = 5 mm in HIV pts (Ann IM 1997;126:123) or pts w pulmonary scars or recent contacts, >10 mm in others; repeat in 2–3 wk to get booster effect, 1/3 more become positive in elderly (Nejm 1985;312:1483) but of questionable significance in the young (Ann IM 1994;120:190); ignore old BCG immunization in interpreting, esp if > 5–10 yr ago; false negs with overwhelming infection, sarcoid, or other anergy; delayed reactivity (IPPD neg at 48 h, pos at 6 d in 25% of SE Asians (Ann IM 1996;124:779)

Urine: Acid, sterile, WBCs and RBCs, protein

Xray: Chest shows apical scarring and/or Ghon complex; IVP characteristically shows beaded ureters

Rx: (Med Let 1992;34:11; Am Rev Resp Dis 1986;134:355)

1st line:

- INH 300 mg qd × 6 mo or b–tiw × 9 mo, with pyridoxine only if >300 mg qd to prevent neuropathy; adverse effect: hepatitis
- Rifampin 600 mg qd or b–tiw × 9 mo, less toxic than streptomycin or INH or longer acting form, rifapentine (Priftin) biw × 2 mos then q wk thereafter (Rx Let 1998;5:46)
- Pyrazinamide 0.5–40 mg/kg/d or b–tiw × 2 mo, with above allows 6-mo cure courses (Am Rev Respir Dis 1991;143:700, 707); rifamate (INH + rifampin) or "Rifater," a combination pill of all 3 (preferable; Ann IM 1995;122:951)

2nd line drugs: ethambutol 15 mg/kg pos qd, use as 4th drug until know sensitivities (Med Let 1995;37–67); adverse effects: retrobulbar neuritis, check visual acuity regularly, rarely reversible

3rd line: streptomycin 250–1000 mg im qd or 20 mg/kg biw

Antibiotic-resistant tbc: 3 drugs to which organism test susceptible × 12–24 mo; frequent now in AIDS pts (Nejm 1993;328:1137; 1992;326:1514; Ann IM 1992;117:177) and infection can be w previously cured strain so must use 4 drugs (Ann IM 1987;106:25)

Prevent:

- Hospital preventive policies (Nejm 1995;332:92) respiratory isolation in negative pressure rooms until 3 negative smears of HIV pts w abnormal chest xray, plus regular skin testing programs (Nejm 1995;332:92; Ann IM 1995;122:658)
- BCG vaccination to entire at-risk population (Jama 1994;271:698); possibly to long-term travelers to areas of high risk (Lancet 2000;356:461)
- INH 300 mg po qd × 9 mo for PPD reactors and household contacts under age 35 (Am J Respir Crit Care Med 2000;161;S221) as well as over 35 if previous neg test or in epidemic (Ann IM 1996;125:114), or perhaps in all since hepatitis risk is small, <1/50,000 die (Ann IM 1997;127:1058); supplement w pyridoxine only if alcoholic and/or malnourished, not for asthmatics on steroids (Ann IM 1976;84:261); in HIV-pos pts w pos PPD

or anergic, 300 mg po qd w B$_6$ (pyridoxine) 50 mg po qd
forever (Lancet 1993;342:268) decr incid by 2/3 at 2 yr
(Nejm 1997;337:801)
- Alternative: rifampin (600 mg d) plus pyrazinamide (25 mg/kg/d)
  × 2 mo, (Am J Respir as above) of active disease (Med Let
  1995;37:67; Ann IM 1990;112:393); contact local health dept,
  use 4 drugs initially in all and continuing in AIDS (Ann IM
  1987;106:25); use tiw directly observed rx for all cases to prevent
  further drug resistance (Jama 1995;274:945; Nejm 1994;330:1179;
  1993;328:576) or biw rx after 2 wk of qd rx; prevalence of drug
  resistance incr from 10% to 36% if take meds for <1 mo
  (Nejm 1998;338:1641)

16.50 TULAREMIA (RABBIT FEVER)

Nejm 1993;329:940

Cause: *Francisella (Pasteurella) tularensis*

Epidem: Worldwide; from infected rodents and lagomorphs, by eating
or handling, or by being bitten by arthropod (tick) vector (50% of
transmissions occur in this way); wherever large rabbit/rodent
populations, eg, muskrats in Vermont; endemic in Martha's
Vineyard, MA, rabbits (Nejm 1979;301:827)

Risk for travelers: Very rare; concern for hunters, mammologists, etc.

Incubation period: 5 d average, but up to 3 wk

Pathophys: Endotoxin production and rapid multiplication, transient
bacteremias lead to all parenchymous organ involvement

Sx: Fever (97%), malaise (60%), headache (23%), nausea and vomiting
(8%), pleuritic chest pain (5%)

Si: Ulcerated papule (94%) at site of entry, very infective; regional
lymphadenopathy (70%); fever and septicemia; Ddx includes
plague (16.32), anthrax (16.1), rickettsial (16.39, 16.41, 16.52),
and more indolent fungal/mycobacterial disease (16.2)

Crs: 2 wk duration on average; 15% relapsc later

Cmplc: Tularemic pneumonia, probably need to inhale to get

Lab:

Bact: Gram-negative bacilli; culture of blood, sputum, or local ulcer
on special medium

Serol: Available from health departments, agglutinin titers

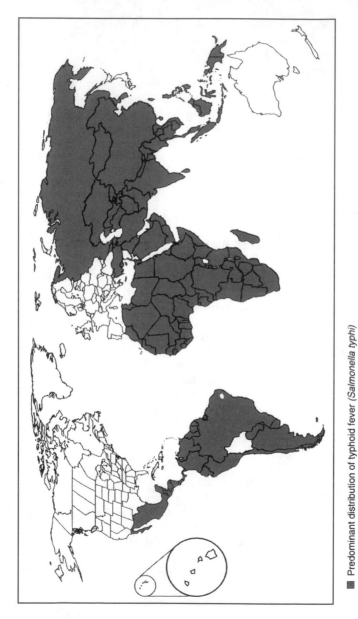

■ Predominant distribution of typhoid fever (*Salmonella typhi*)

Figure 16.3. Predominant distribution of typhoid fever (*salmonella typhi*). (Reproduced with permission from Tropical Infectious Diseases.)

Rx: 1st choice, streptomycin 1 gm im qd × 14 d, or gentamicin; 2nd, tetracycline or chloramphenicol
Prevent: avoid tick bites, contact w wild animals

16.51 TYPHOID (ENTERIC) FEVER

Inf Contr Hosp Epidem 1991;12:168; JAMA 1997;278:847; Guerrant Trop Inf Dis, 1st ed, 1999:277

Cause: *Salmonella typhi*

Epidem: 16 million cases/yr worldwide; 2/3 cases from Asia, 1/3 Africa; endemic in Indian subcontinent, Africa, Central and South America; mortality rates 12–32% in developing countries (see Fig. 16.3)

Fecal–oral vehicles may include fruit, raw vegetables, shellfish; no natural reservoir except human carriers (2–3% of recovered population), probably resides in gallbladder

Increased incidence in U.S. foreign travelers, cirrhotics, patients with tumors esp of CNS, hemolytic anemias esp sickle cell anemia, aortic aneurysms esp thoracic

Risk for travelers: 300 cases confirmed in U.S./yr; 80% associated w travel outside U.S. (Jama 2000;283:2668); greatest in U.S. travelers returning from Indian subcontinent (57%); 6% from Mexico; risk is low (from 1 to 800 per million travelers to various low-income countries) (Arch IM 1998;158:663) but incr w adventure travel, adoption of local dietary habits, persons visiting families

Pathophys: Endotoxin production; intracellular organisms; ingestion results in infection of mesenteric lymph nodes via macrophages that release active cytokines, include TNF, il-1, others; spread throughout reticuloendothelial system w nodes' subsequent necrosis over 2 wk, leading to septicemia and further node, involvement plus ulceration

Incubation period: 6–22 d

Sx: Fever >38.5°C (100°F); abdominal pain (20–40%), constipation (10–38%), rarely diarrhea; also may have headache, cough, sore throat, dizziness, confusion, or psychosis (5%)

Si: Fever (100%), bradycardia P < 100 (40–80%), splenomegaly (50–75%), hepatomegaly (30%), salmon-colored macular rash (rose spots) over lower chest (5–30%); may have cervical lymphadenopathy; jaundice w incr AST (10%), sometimes w encephalopathy c/w fulminant liver failure (Mayo Clin Proc 2000;75:462)

Crs: Fever gradually up, then gradually down over days, even with rx

Cmplc: Usually occur in third–fourth week; mortality even with rx especially if septicemia; relapse (10%); metastatic infections to lung, brain, joints, aorta (10%); intestinal hemorrhage (7%); intestinal perforation (3%); pneumonia and/or multiple pulmonary emboli; delerium, coma; other neurologic complications may include meningitis, encephalomyelitis, spastic paraparesis, cranial neuritis, ascending paralysis; acute cholecystitis (1–2%), glomerulonephritis (1%)

Lab:

Bact: blood culture, 50–80% positive in 1st 2 wk; bone marrow 90% sensitive (26% positive even when blood negative); culture of bx rose spots (60%); stool culture (30% but rises up to 80% after 1 wk); Gram's stain shows gram-negative rods; stool mucus methylene blue stain shows WBCs, mostly mononuclear unlike polys of salmonellosis, shigellosis, and ulcerative colitis (Ann IM 1972;76:697)

Serol: Widal's test positive after 2 wk, seldom used now (sens 50–90%, spec 50–70%)

DNA probes and PCR: increase specificity (flagellin based, 90% sens, nearly 100% spec)

Rx: Note incr prev of multidrug resistant strains (Jama 2000;283:2668)

- Ciprofloxacin, other quinolones (cure rates nearly 100%); recent rx failures (Lancet 1999;353:1590); or
- Chloramphenicol 4 g qd × 4 wk; 15 g/d when acute; or 15 g qd × 14 d (Nejm 1968;278:171), some resistance (Nejm 1973;289:463); cure rates 90% w sensitive strains
- Ampicillin as good as chloro although some R plasmid-mediated resistance too (Nejm 1969;280:147)
- Tm/S (Nejm 1980;303:426)
- Cephalosporins, 3rd generation

Delirium leading to coma and/or shock: dexamethasone 3 mg/kg × 1, then 1 mg/kg q 6 h × 48 h, decreases mortality from 55% to 10% (Nejm 1984;310:82)

Prevent:
- Keep carriers out of food, water; chlorinate water; treat carriers; ampicillin 6 g qd with 2 g probenecid (Med Let 1968;10:51), or ciprofloxacin 500 mg bid × 28 d (Nejm 1991;324:392) for carriers; if no response, cholecystectomy is effective
- Immunize (Med Let 1994;36:41) with live attenuated Ty21a vaccine (Vivotif) po qod × 4 beginning at least 2 wk before departure, good for 5 yr; or capsular polysaccharide vaccine (Typhim Vi) im × 1, ~80% effective (see Chapter 3)

16.52 TYPHUS

Cause: *Rickettsia prowazekii* and *mooseri, R. typhi*

Epidem: Worldwide; endemic: human-to-human via human body louse or lab technique (Ann IM 1968;69:731); worldwide; especially winter/spring in cold climates

Brill–Zinsser disease: recurrent disease in carriers, perhaps via fleas

Murine type: human to rat to human

Risk to travelers: Rare

Pathophys: Arteritis by intracellular invasion causing vascular occlusion. Nodules in cortical gray matter

Incubation Period: 10 d

Sx: Headache; rash (can abort with early rx; Ann IM 1968;69:731)

Si: Fever; rash, centrifugal (central body spreading to extremities); pneumonia, atypical; CNS sx; necrotic skin over pressure points

Crs: Variable; self-limited in 2–3 wks; sometimes fatal

Cmplc: May precipitate GGPD deficiency in blacks, leading to hemolysis and subsequent ATN (Ann IM 1968;69:323)

Lab:
Chem: LFTs show hepatitis picture (Ann IM 1968;69:731)
Serol: Weil–Felix OX19 positive (r/o RMSF and scrub typhus)

Rx: Tetracycline or chloramphenicol; loading dose 2–2.5 × daily dose, then rx × 10 d

Prevent: Kill lice with DDT; kill rats

16.53 YERSINIA GASTROENTERITIS

Nejm 1989;321:16

Cause: *Yersinia enterocolitica*

Epidem: Fecal–oral; associated with poor sanitation; can live and reproduce at 4°C, hence can occur in winter too; animal reservoirs, especially pigs (Nejm 1990;322:984); contaminated chocolate milk in NY school epidemic (Nejm 1978;298:76); meat and milk products, fecally contaminated water; person-to-person transmission rare, but can occur especially w blood transfusions

Risk for travelers: = domestic risk, but may be incr in northern climates (ie, Scandinavia)

Pathophys: Bowel wall invasion

Sx: Headache, sore throat, fever (FUO occasionally), abdominal pain, chronic and recurrent diarrhea

Si: Exudative pharyngitis especially in adults (Ann IM 1983;99:40), fever, erythema nodosum, polyarthritis (Bull Rheum Dis 1979;29:100)

Crs: 2^+ wk, even with antibiotic rx

Cmplc: Misdiagnosed as appendicitis and as regional enteritis (Nejm 1990;323:113); massive GI bleed or perforation; thyrotoxicosis (Ann IM 1976;85:735); bacteremia, esp if iron overloaded, which fuels growth, 50% fatal; postinfectious arthropathy (HLA B27-associated) r/o other more common forms of gastroenteritis (NV + D), such as viral, esp from "small round-structured viruses" (Jama 1997;278:563)

Lab:

Bact: Gram-negative rod, an enterobacteriaceae; grows best at 25°C in 24–48 h; facultative anaerobe

Serol: Passive hemagglutinin titer >1/512 diagnostic but 30% false negatives

Rx: Questionable that rx helps uncomplicated cases; in patients with focal, extraintestinal infections or bacteremia: 1st gentamicin + doxycycline pending sensitivities; fluoroquinolones, maybe chloramphenicol or tetracyclines alone

Prevent: Avoid unpasteurized dairy products

17 Fungal Disease

17.1 BLASTOMYCOSIS

Nejm 1986;314:529, 575

Cause: *Blastomyces dermatitidis*

Epidem: Primarily U.S., river valleys from Minn to Mississippi; endemic focus also in So Africa (Rev Inf Dis 1991;13:1005); scattered foci also worldwide; Airborne in rotten wood dust; No America esp around the Great Lakes and southeastern U.S.; occasional large outbreaks due to soil exposure

Risk for travelers: Rare (= local U.S. risk)

Pathophys: Inhalation of spores leads to pneumonia, then possible dissemination

Incubation period: 3–12 wk

Sx: Asx (50%), cough (45%), ha (32%), chest pain (30%), weight loss (28%), fever (25%)

Si: Nodular or ulcerative skin lesions

Crs: Usually self-limited, 3–4 wk (Nejm 1974;290:540)

Cmplc: Chronic infection involves lungs (cavitary), skin, prostate, bones; rare in AIDS pts, but CNS involved when infection does occur; r/o South American blastomycosis (paracoccidioidomycosis), which is transmitted by thorn pricks and causes skin disease that looks like leprosy (see 17.6)

Lab:

   Bact: diphasic but yeast form in tissue; braziliensis has multiple budding in yeast form

   Serol: CF antibodies positive in only 10% (Nejm 1974;290:540); immunodiffusion positive in 28% of true positives; enzyme immunoassay positive in 77%

   Skin test: doubtful usefulness, positive in <40% proven cases (Am Rev Respir Dis 1988;138:1081; Nejm 1986;314:529, 575)

Xray: Positive chest xray if pulmonic

Rx: Amphotericin, or itraconazole 400 mg qd po × 6 mo (Am J Med 1992;93:489); ampho B (low dose) results in 80% cure; high dose results in 100% cure but 60% side effects (Ann IM 1985;103:861, 872); ampho not for meningitis; perhaps itraconazole

17.2 COCCIDIOIDOMYCOSIS

Nejm 1995;332:1077

Cause: *Coccidioides immitis*

Epidem: No and So American desert (Lower Sonoran) regions; see Fig. 17.1; airborne spread (inhalation) of mycelial stage infective spores; endospore spread in body (description of storm-scattered epidemic in California; Nejm 1979;301:358); American southwest esp Arizona, Texas, and Calif, eg, San Joaquin valley (Stockton to Bakersfield); also parts of Mexico, Venezuela, Honduras, Guatemala, Patagonia; worst in wet season, esp in patients exposed to dirt in spring and late fall; increased risk dissemination in pregnancy, Asians, African Americans, and patients on steroid rx, in AIDS, and other

Risk for travelers: Low; but increased for archeologists, biologists, others w contact w soil working in endemic areas; recent outbreak among U.S. volunteers constructing a church in Mexico (Mmwr 2000;49:1001)

Incubation period: 1–3 wk; 40% develop sx; reactivation w AIDS yrs later

Sx: Hemoptysis; granulomatous reactions of face and neck; primary cocci picture (Nejm 1972;286:507) of pneumonitis (Nejm 1970;283:325), flu-like syndrome with generalized pruritus, macular/papular rash; ha; acute polyarthritis (Nejm 1972;287:1133)

Si: Erythema nodosum, pleural effusion

Crs: Mortality 1% in Caucasians, 20% in Asians and Mexicans with disseminated disease; recurrent up to 10 yr after amphotericin rx (Nejm 1969;281:950)

Cmplc: Hypercalcemia (Nejm 1977;297:431); dissemination in 0.5–1% w extrapulmonary lesions, onset 1+ yr after primary pulmonary infection (eg, bones, joints, skin, meninges)

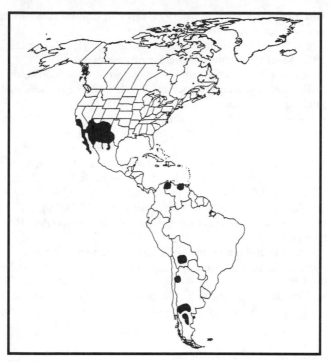

Coccidioidomycosis

Figure 17.1. Distribution of *coccidioides immitis.* (Reproduced with permission from Tropical Infectious Diseases.)

Lab:

    Bact: mycelial form (white, fluffy, distinctive) dangerous to lab personnel; diphasic but no yeast forms in tissue; urine culture frequently positive if concentrated by lab, even when do not suspect disseminated disease; prostate secretion culture also often positive in same circumstances (Ann IM 1976;85:34)

    Serol: Several tests including tube precipitation test (IgM); EIA (IgM, IgG), comp-fix antibody titer >1/16 suggests disseminated active disease; positive in 14/15 (Nejm 1970;283:326); decreases with successful rx; counterimmunoelectrophoresis titer has 8%

Fungal Disease **179**

false-negative rate (Ann IM 1976;85:740); CSF ID comp-fix test pos is diagnostic of coccidial meningitis

Skin test: 20–50% false neg but still useful (Am Rev Respir Dis 1988;138:1081); indicates present or past disease

Xray: Nodular pneumonitis; primary pneumonias; coin lesions; thin-walled cavities, hilar adenopathy; r/o rheumatoid nodules and pneumatoceles; sarcoid; tbc

Rx: Beware steroids; meningitis after acute rx must be rx w lifelong suppression (Ann IM 1996;124:305) of acute disease (Nejm 1987;317:334):

- Amphotericin 1 to 1.5 mg/kg iv 2×/wk to total of 30 mg/kg if sick, if comp-fix is increased, or if hx of and on steroids; 20% relapse (4/20; Nejm 1970;283:325); intrathecal for meningitis, many complications especially with reservoir (Nejm 1973;288:186)
- Fluconazole po × yr effectively suppresses meningitis (Ann IM 1993;119:28)
- Itraconazole 200 mg po bid is effective; recent studies favor itraconazole, fluconazole as first line rx (Am J Med 1990;89:292; also 1995;98:249)

Prevent: Travelers engaging in high-exposure activities in endemic areas should consider use of particle filter mask during excavations, etc.

17.3 CRYPTOCOCCOSIS

Rev Inf Dis 1991;13:1163; Ann IM 1981;94:611

Cause: *Cryptococcus neoformans*

Epidem: Worldwide; ubiquitous fungus; airborne; birds are probable vectors, esp pigeons, grows well in bird guano; Australian var (*C. neoformans gatti*) assoc w eucalyptus trees, causes severe pneumonia/meningitis in immunocompetent pts; increased incidence of all varieties of cryptococcus in patients with lymphomas and/or on steroids, AIDS

Risk in travelers: Rare (= domestic risk); possible increased risk in Australia or other areas w endemic *C. neoformans* var. *gatti*

Pathophys: Dissemination in pts w decr cell-mediated immunity to lungs, CNS, skin

Incubation period: days to weeks

Sx: Meningitis, pneumonitis (Am Rev Respir Dis 1966;94:236)

Si: altered mental status; rare papilledema w obstructive hydrocephalus

Crs: Without rx, nearly 100% dead in 1 yr; with rx, 70% survival, 18% relapse in 29 mo (Ann IM 1969;71:1079) (review of good and bad prognosis test results; Ann IM 1974;80:176)

Cmplc: Renal papillary necrosis (Nejm 1968;279:60); resistant prostatitis despite rx (Ann IM 1989;111:125)

Lab:

Bact: Smear sputum, CSF, urine; round nucleoli, large nonstaining capsule, looks like lymphocyte; India ink preparation (drop of ink to CSF) reveals large clear (large capsules) organisms but 35% can have CNS crypto and neg India ink prep (NIH-Ann IM 1969;71:1079); culture yeast form on rice/Tween agar at 22° and 37°C; need large volumes of CSF to find

Serol: Antigen by latex fixation or comp-fix is the only clinically useful test; antigen in bronchopulmonary lavage fluid 100% sens, 98% specif (Am Rev Respir Dis 1992;145:226); sens also high in serum or CSF; antibody, by indirect fluorescent antibody (IFA); 92% patients positive for one or the other in CSF and/or serum (Nejm 1977;297:1440); patients with positive antigen levels do more poorly; false-positive IFA in 2% normals, 6% blastos, 12% histos; no false-positive antigen tests; hence rx a positive antigen but not a positive IFA (Ann IM 1968;69:1113, 1117)

Skin test: False positive in 31%; interferes with serologic testing (Ann IM 1968;69:45)

Xray: CT scan for mass lesions in head, which will decrease with medical rx (Ann IM 1981;94:382); occasional pulmonary nodules

Rx:

• Amphotericin B 2–2.5 g total course, 0.3–0.7 mg/kg iv qd (Nejm 1997;337:15); no proven advantage in intrathecal use (Ann IM 1969;71:1079), lots of complications especially with reservoir for intrathecal use (Nejm 1973;288:186)

• Adjunct w ampho B: 5-flucytosine 50–150 mg/kg/d po qid (Ann IM 1977;86:318; Nejm 1974;290:320); hematologic toxicity; use with amphotericin to prevent resistance and vs meningeal disease ×6 wk (Nejm 1979;301:126) or occasionally 4 wk in otherwise healthy (Nejm 1987;317:334); in AIDS meningitis rx w amphotericin and flucytosine ×2 wk then fluconazole or itraconazole maintenance (Nejm 1997;337:15; 1989;321:794)

FUNGAL DISEASE

- Fluconazole or itraconazole as good as and less toxic than amphotericin in AIDS patients with meningitis (Nejm 1992;326:83, 793); maintenance postepisode prevents recurrence in AIDS patients (Nejm 1997;337:15; 1991;324:580)

17.4 HISTOPLASMOSIS

Cause: *Histoplasma capsulatum* (in W hemisphere; var. *duboisii* in Africa)

Epidem: North and South America; tropical Africa (var. *duboisii*); see Fig. 17.2; bats and birds vectors via airborne spores; frequently in rolling green countryside (opposite of cocci) (eg, Ohio Valley; Ann IM 1981;94:331, 100,000 patient outbreak in Indianapolis)

Risk for travelers: Low, but incr in spelunkers, others w unusual exposure (ie, biologists, etc.); recent large (>200 tourists) outbreak in Mexico (Mmwr 2001;50:261)

Pathophys: Intracellular; 3 clinical syndromes:
- Acute primary (pulmonary)
- Chronic cavitary (pulmonary)
- Progressive disseminated (Ann IM 1972;76:557)

Incubation period: days to yrs

Sx: Pulmonary, acute immune complex-type polyarthritis

Si: Chorioretinitis, focal, macular choroid inflammation, and hemorrhage without vitreous reaction (present with all other types of chorioretinitis); hepatomegaly; erythema nodosum

Crs: Usually benign

Cmplc:
- Fibrosing syndromes of mediastinum and/or retroperitoneum
- Endocarditis (rare)
- Adrenal insufficiency in 50% of disseminated form (Ann IM 1971;75:511)
- Meningitis, chronic, like cryptococcus
- Ulcerative enteritis, esp of distal ileum and colon; var. *duboisii* (Africa); chronic skin, bone disease

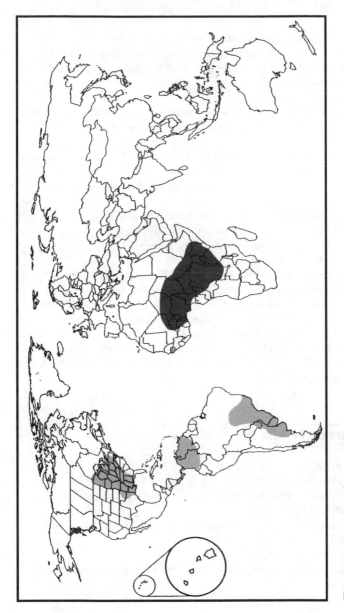

■ American histoplasmosis

■ African histoplasmosis

Figure 17.2. Distribution of *histoplasma capsulatum*. (Reproduced with permission from Tropical Infectious Diseases.)

Lab:

Bact: silver stain demonstrates; cannot see with H + E or Giemsa; culture of liver, marrow, nodes; positive in ~20% (Ann IM 1982;97:680); slow grower, takes >2 wk; filamentous strands of hyphal sporangia; distinctive chlamydospores when grown at room temperature

Hem: anemia, thrombocytopenia; marrow culture and stain positive

Serol: (Ann IM 1982;97:680): comp-fix antibody titer positive in 96% of patients with active, disseminated disease; immunodiffusion antibody titer positive in 87%; RIA for antigen positive in urine (90%) and blood (50%) in disseminated disease (Nejm 1986;314:83) and more accurate than antibody titers (Ann IM 1991;115:936)

Skin test: many false positives and negatives, interferes with serologic testing (Am Rev Respir Dis 1964;90:927)

Xray: "Buckshot" calcifications in lungs, spleen

Rx: Steroids for choroid infections

Usual Rx: Itraconazole (400 mg/d, then 200 mg/d × 6 mo; Am J Med 1992;93:489); alternative, amphotericin 1/2 mg/kg iv × 2/wk to a total of 35–40 mg/kg initial course (Ann IM 1971;75:511); use prophylactically if past hx and starting steroids (Nejm 1969;280:206), or if patient has AIDS and has been rx to cure (Ann IM 1989;111:655) or, ketoconazole, 400 mg qd po × 6 mo cures 85% all types (Ann IM 1985;103:861) even cavitary disease but not meningitis

17.5 MYCETOMA

Guerrant Trop Inf Dis 1999; ch 59

Cause: Soil fungi and actinomycetes

Epidem: Tropics/subtropics worldwide; rural workers—risk assoc w barefoot work

Risk for travelers: Not reported to occur w usual travel; cases in U.S. usually seen in refugee populations

Incubation period: Variable (wk–mo)

Pathophys: Invasion of soft tissues, bone by fungal or actinomycotic species

Sx: Nodule develops w sinus/fistula; discharges purulent material—
grains/granules; most on lower extremities but may occur on
hands
Si: Swelling, w fistulae; regional lymphadenopathy
Crs: Chronic swelling, soft tissue/bone destruction
Dx: Stain and culture IMPERATIVE to determine causative organisms
Rx: Depends upon species present; ie rx differs for
nocardia/actinomycetes vs soil fungi; surgical debridement
decreases duration of antibiotic rx
Prevent: Use of footwear

17.6 PARACOCCIDIOIDOMYCOSIS ("SOUTH AMERICAN BLASTOMYCOSIS")

Guerrant et al; Trop Inf Dis 1999; ch 62
Cause: *Paracoccidioides brasiliensis*
Epidem: Mexico, Central and So America; see Fig. 17.3; assoc w
rainforest areas; rural workers (ie, woodcutters) are at most risk;
recent incr in disseminated disease assoc w incr in HIV
Risk for travelers: Very rare
Incubation period: Latency for 15 yr
Sx: cough, wght loss
Si: lymphadenopathy, hepatosplenomegaly, skin/mucosal ulcerative
lesions
Crs:
Juvenile—disseminates to multiple sites; this form predominant in pts
w HIV
Adult—progressive pulmonary disease (90%)
Dx: Potassium iodide stain of sputum: tissue bx w characteristic "pilot
wheel" appearance; culture in Sabouraud's media
Rx: Options include sulfadiazine, Tm/S, and imidazoles; itraconazole is
currently preferred (CID 1999;28:947)
Prevent: Prophylaxis w Tm/S for PCP in HIV pts may also have effect
on paracoccidioidomycosis (CID 1999;28:947)

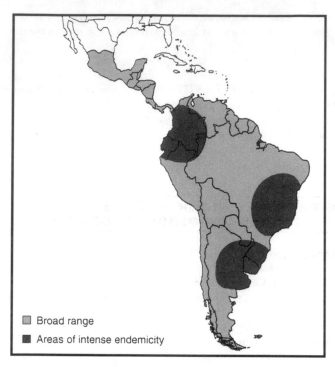

Figure 17.3. Distribution of *paracoccidioides brasiliensis.* (Reproduced with permission from Tropical Infectious Diseases.)

Broad range

Areas of intense endemicity

17.7 PENICILLIOSIS

CID 1999;28:947

Cause: *Penicillium marneffei*, a dimorphic fungus

Epidem: Endemic to SE Asia, So China; a rare cause of disease until AIDS epidemic; affect up to 1/4 of AIDS pts in No Thailand; exposure to soil, especially during rainy season a risk; reservoir may include bamboo rat

Risk for travelers: Very rare, but a consideration in persons w AIDS w prolonged travel/residence planned in endemic areas

Incubation period: Unknown; most cases appear to be due to reactivation; but may develop disseminated disease w/i wk of exposure

Sx: Fever, weight loss, cough, rash

Si: Fever; cutaneous lesions, including papular rash w central umbilication (as w molluscum contagiosum), on face, scalp, upper extremities, elsewhere; also may have maculopapular rash, sc nodules; may occur w/o rash, w hepatic involvement as major si

Crs: Progressive decline w high mortality if not treated

Lab: Anemia; incr alk phos common

Path: Typical intra- and extracellular yeast like organisms on lymph node or bone marrow aspirate, or touch prep of skin; culture of blood (76%), skin bx (90%), bone marrow (100%) all sensitive

Rx: Amphotericin B (0.6 mg/kg/d) × several wks; eventual switch to itraconazole (200 mg bid)

17.8 SPOROTRICHOSIS

Nejm 1994;331:181

Cause: *Sporothrix schenckii*

Epidem: Prick from infected plant, on which are saprophytes, or inhalation; worldwide; esp Mexico, Africa, Latin America; gardeners, farmers, basket makers especially prone; in U.S., large outbreak assoc w sphagnum moss

Risk for travelers: Low; presumably a risk for ecotourists, adventure travelers w direct soil/vegetation contact

Pathophys: Biphasic fungus, mold in wild, yeast in body

Sx: Pustule at contact point w development of nodule and then secondary lesions; usually w/o systemic sx

Si: Peripheral lesion with nodular lymphangitis, or, in inhalation type, pulmonary or systemic sx (Ann IM 1970;73:23) resulting in suppurative arthritis (Ann IM 1977;86:294), multiple skin nodules

Crs: Extracutaneous sites in 1/4

Cmplc: Chronic meningitis (Nejm 1987;317:935); r/o (Ann IM 1993;119:883) tularemia (especially in hunters), nocardia, leishmania, *Mycobacterium marinum, Pseudomonas pseudomallei*, histo, cocci, blasto

Lab:

Bact: Diphasic, but yeast form (cigar shape) is arranged in asteroid bodies in tissue; culture at 22°C results in leathery distinctive mycelial growth

Serol: CF titer = 1/8 in systemic (not cutaneous) disease

Rx: Itraconazole; alternative is potassium iodide (KI) + iodine (I_2) (SSKI) 3 cc qd, increased to 9–12 cc qd (Nejm 1974;290:320); amphoterin B for rare treatment resistant cases; heat rx of cutaneous lesions has been effective, surgical resection of pulmonary cavities

18 Parasitic Disease

18.1 AFRICAN SLEEPING SICKNESS (TRYPANOSOMIASIS)

Ann IM 1977;86:633; Lancet 1996;348:1427

Cause: *Trypanosoma gambiense, T. rhodesiense*

Epidem: SubSaharan and Central Africa, also Botswana, parts of So Africa (endemic from 14 deg north to 15 deg south); see Fig. 18.1; 2 forms; W African (Gambian) in villages along rivers; E African; in savannah areas

Via tsetse fly (*Glossina* sp) from ungulate or human reservoir; inoculation through bite of fly, local multiplication, parasitemia in 3 wk

Risk for travelers: Very rare (1–2 cases per year in U.S., usually w intensive game park exposure to tsetse flies); most in U.S. tourists have been E African form; flies are day-time biters, attracted to moving vehicles (ie, safari vans, etc.)

Pathophys: Vascular cuffing and obliteration in CNS; destruction of lymph nodes leading to fibrosis

Incubation period: Acute symptoms, 5 d to several wk for *T. rhodesiense*, mo to yr for *T. gambiense*; 80% of U.S. cases presented w/i 14 d of tsetse bites

Sx: Fever, weight loss, somnolence, painless nodule at site of bite (often 1 cm or more diameter)

Si: Edema of face, etc.; hyperesthesia; splenomegaly; lymphadenopathy, esp postcerv = Winterbottom's si; rash, often circinate; painless chancre (1–2 wk after bite) subsides in 2 to 3 mo

Crs: Virulent (fatal in days), to chronic (mo–yr)

Cmplc: Encephalitis w apathy (esp frontal lobes, pons, medulla) and somnolence punctuated by intermittent mania; Ddx includes rabies, other viral enceph, etc.

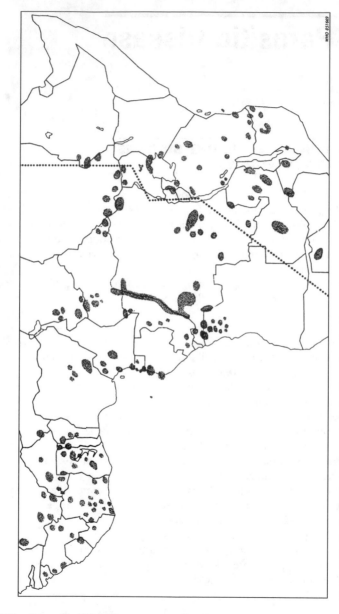

Figure 18.1. Foci of African trypanosomiasis. (Reproduced with permission from WHO, *Epidemiology and control of trypanosomiasis*, WHO Technical Report Series 739.)

Lab:

Hem and CSF: wet smear shows many polymorphic, squirming organisms; trypanosomes also identified in tissue (Wright's stain) from chancre, lymph node, bone marrow; can culture (axenic or animal)

Serol: comp-fix or agglutination antibody elevations (false pos common)

Rx: Contact CDC; early disease: suramin, eflornithine (*T. gambiense* only); late disease: melarsoprol (assoc w reactive enceph in 18%); eflornithine; (for *T. gambiense* only); tryparsamide plus suramin (for T. rhodesiense)

Prevent: Insect repellants may not be effective; flies can pierce light clothing; use dull-colored medium weight clothing in risk areas; for long-term residence, use w insecticide, clear brush around homes; prophylaxis w suramin or pentamidine, but risk of disease is less than the toxicity of drugs (Ann IM 1972;77:797)

18.2 AMEBIASIS

Nejm 1984;310:298; 1978;298:262; Ann IM 1996;124:429

Cause: *Entamoeba histolytica, Entamoeba dispar* (usually nonpathogenic), *Dientamoeba fragilis*; note that several NONPATHOGENS may be reported on stool O + P, incl *Endolimax nana, Entamoeba coli, Iodoamoeba butschlii*

Epidem: Worldwide; most pathogenic species (*E. histolytica*) common in tropics; encysted organisms excreted in feces, contaminates water or food; human carriers disseminate; degree of infestation correlates inversely with sanitation

Risk for travelers: Low incidence in short-term travelers; but over 50% Peace Corps volunteers in India developed amebiasis in 2-yr stint (Wilson, 1991)

Pathophys: Trophozoite (amoebic form) invades wall of colon, secretes autolyzing enzymes, and lives on necrotic tissue in abscess; multiplies by binary fission

Incubation period: Colitis: 1–3 wk; amebic liver abcess: 2 wk to several mo

Sx: Fever, bloody stool, alternating diarrhea and constipation; most cases are mild, but dysenteric in 10% *E. histolytica*; asymptomatic cyst passers are common, esp with *E. dispar*

Si: RUQ abdom tenderness

Crs: Usually self-limited over 1–4 wk, but chronic relapsing disease can occur

Cmplc: Abscess metastases to liver, lung, brain, pericardium, spleen, skin (ulcers); pain, abnl LFTs, often without diarrhea; r/o the much more benign, CILIATE DYSENTERY caused by *Balantidium coli*, and nonpathogenic strains of *E. histolytica*—now designated *E. dispar*—which are commensals in gay males, institutionalized individuals (Nejm 1986;315:353, 390); *E. dispar* can only be distinguished from *E. histolytica* by antigen detection; note also lab reports of *Entamoeba coli*, *Endolimax nana* represent bowel commensal nonpathogens

Lab:

Serol: Elevated antibody titers, 90% sensitive (Ann IM 1969;71:983) for extraintestinal disease; 80% sensitive for invasive colonic disease

Stool: O + P positive in 90% with severe colonic disease; 3 stools are 70% sensitive with mild disease; cysts with 4 nuclei, central nucleolus; often overdiagnosed by lab technicians thinking WBCs are ameba (Ann IM 1978;88:89); recogniton of need to distinguish *E. dispar* from *E. histolytica* makes stool antigen detection tests preferable to O + P exams

Stool antigen tests show good sensitivity (87%) and can distinguish *E. histolytica* from *E. dispar* (Techlabs)

Xray: BE shows deformed cecum, narrowed; rarely megacolon

Rx: asymptomatic cyst passer (*E. histolytica*): iodoquinol 650 mg or 10 mg/kg po tid × 20 d; or paromomycin 8–10 mg/kg po tid × 7 d or dilanoxide furorate (available from CDC; CID 1992;15:464); of intestinal disease: metronidazole 10–12 mg/kg or 750 mg po tid × 10 d; or tinidazole 50 mg/kg up to 2 gm/d × 3–5 d plus iodoquinol or paromomycin or dilanoxide; of hepatic abscess: metronidazole as above; or tinidazole 800 mg tid × 5 d

Prevent: Tetraglycine hydroperiodate kills cysts in 30 min; boiling effective; chlorination less effective

18.3 AMEBIC MENINGOENCEPHALITIS

Ann IM 1978;88:468

Cause: *Naegleria gruberi, N. fowleri*

Epidem: Worldwide, particularly warm climates; natural inhabitant of freshwater; in patients (usually children) who have been swimming in past week; very rare

Risk for travelers: Very rare

Pathophys: Meningoencephalitis with predilection for olfactory, cerebellar, and temporofrontal areas; later develop hematogenous spread and often fatal myocarditis; may invade via nose through cribriform plate and into olfactory bulb

Incubation period: 1–2 wk

Sx: Headache, swam within past week, fever (*Acanthamoeba* can also cause ocular keratitis in contact lens wearers)

Si: Parosmia (funny smells), cerebellar ataxia, meningoencephalitis without increased CNS pressure

Crs: Almost universally fatal in 4–5 d

Cmplc: Death

Lab:

CSF: purulent meningitis with "bubbly" ameba on high-power wet mount

Path: organisms in all organs but gi tract

Rx: A few survivors now (Nejm 1982;306:346; Ann IM 1971;74:923); amphotericin B iv and perhaps intracisternally; perhaps ketoconazole, or flucytosine; 1 case disseminated acanthameba cured w pentamidine (Nejm 1994;331:88); of keratitis: topical 0.1% propamidine + neosporin; or itraconazole po + topical miconazole

Prevent: Avoid warm (>32°C) swimming holes/ponds, esp w apparent coliform contamination

18.4 ANISAKIASIS (INTESTINAL)

Jama 1985;253:1012

Cause: Anisakis larva (fish nematodes) of several species

Epidem: Worldwide; most common in Japan, Europe where fish are often eaten raw; worms live in fish viscera, but may migrate to muscles if fish not filleted promptly; occurs with numerous species including herring, cod, mackerel, squid

Risk for travelers: Rarely reported (no risk w dietary avoidance of raw fish)

Incubation period: 12–48 hr to wk for intestinal

Pathophys: Local inflammatory response at site of larval penetration of GI tract (stomach, small intestine, colon)

Sx: Abdominal pain, nausea, vomiting, usually within 12–24 hr of ingestion; intestinal may mimic appendicitis

Si: Sometimes peritonitis

Crs: Usually self-limited, but intestinal penetration can lead to chronic inflammation consistent with regional enteritis

Complc: Peritonitis secondary to bowel perforation, GI bleeding

Dx: Endoscopy or surgical removal of larvae

Rx: Usually conservative management; extraction by endoscopy, surgery has been successful

Prevent: Fillet fresh fish; cook to 60°C for 10 min or freeze 24 hr at −20°C

18.5 ANGIOSTRONGYLIASIS (MENINGITIS AND GASTROINTESTINAL)

Nejm 1995;332:1105

Cause: Rat lung worms; *Angiostrongylus cantonensis* (eosinophilic meningitis), *A. costaricensis* (eosinophilic gastroenteritis)

Epidem: *A. cantonensis*: spread from Asia to ports around the world by infected rats; infection of humans from ingestion of larval worms from raw or marinated snails (Thai delicacy = pila snails), slugs, or possibly undercooked vegetables contaminated by snails

A. costaricensis: So Mexico to Argentina; most case reports from Costa Rica; cotton rat–snail cycle; infection from contaminated plants (recent outbreak linked to mint; CID 1998;26:365)

Risk to travelers: Very rare, but recent outbreak of eosinophilic meningitis in group of tourists to Jamaica consistent with incr spread of vector snails

Incubation period: 2 wk for meningitis (*A. cantonensis*), 2–4 wk for abd (*A. costaricensis*)

Pathophys: Larval migration w eosinophilic inflammation, granulomatous arteritis

Sx: *A. cantonensis*: severe ha, fever, asymmetric paresthesias, transient CN palsies

 A. costaricensis: fever, nausea, abd pain (mimics appendicitis)

Si: As above

Crs: Most are self-limited (2–8 wk for meningitis); deaths have been reported

Lab: *Hem*: eosinophilia, leukocytosis common w both; in menigitis, CSF eos are common (use Wright's stain on CSF)

Dx: Serology available from CDC for *A. cantonensis*

Rx: Prednisone may have benefit for CNS disease

Prevent: Avoid unwashed vegetables, raw or marinated snails

18.6 ASCARIASIS AND TRICHURIASIS (WHIPWORM)

Nejm 1984;310:298

Cause:

 Ascariasis: *Ascaris lumbricoides*, pig roundworm

 Trichuriasis: *Trichuris trichiura*

Epidem: Worldwide; highest incidence of both is in tropics, where eggs survive more easily, and in children who do more fecal–oral transmission

 Ascariasis: fecal–oral, 2 wk incubation of eggs necessary outside body before infective; eggs can remain infective in moist soil for years

 Trichuriasis: fecal–oral

Risk for travelers: Rare; domestic risk (U.S.) in gardeners using animal feces for fertilizer

Incubation period: Days to wks

Pathophys: Larval migration of Ascaris causes hypersensitivity
pneumonitis

Sx:

Ascariasis: only if abnormal site or so many that they block GI tract;
after ingestion, migrate to lungs, then coughed up, reingested

Trichuriasis: embed in superficial intestinal mucosa, mainly colon;
no tissue reaction, hence occasionally diarrhea

Si: Usually none

Crs: Lifespan of worm (Ascaris) is 10–24 mo

Cmplc:

Ascariasis: small bowel obstruction; perforated bowel; asphyxia due
to aspiration; biliary obstruction; hepatic abscess

Trichuriasis: anemia, malnutrition; rectal prolapse; allergic
pneumonitis (in 10%)

Lab:

Bact:

Ascariasis: stool shows eggs, and adults

Trichuriasis: stool shows barrel-shaped eggs w mucous plug at both
ends; adults, whip is head end, handle is tail end

Rx: (Nejm 1996;334:1178)

- Mebendazole (Vermox) 100 mg bid × 3 d, or
- Albendazole (400 mg single dose for Ascaris, × 3 d for trichuris), or
- Ivermectin, piperazine, pyrantel pamoate are alternatives for Ascaris

Prevent: Avoid reinfection; worms live <2 yr

18.7 BABESIOSIS

Nejm 1993;329:943; 1977;297:825; CID 2001;32:1117

Cause: *Babesia microti; also B. divergens*, B. strain WA-1

Epidem: Several species worldwide; most cases reported from U.S.
and Europe; transmitted by ticks of cattle, mice, and deer or by
transfusion of infected blood (Ann IM 1982;96:601); endemic
in Nantucket, Fire Island NY, coastal New England, Georgia,
Mexico, California (Nejm 1995;332:298), Missouri (Ann IM
124;643–650), Washington State (Ann IM 1993;119:284);
Europe (*B. divergens*); incidence of symptomatic disease/severe
disease increased in AIDS and splenectomized patients
(Nejm 1980;303:1098)

Risk for travelers: Focally high risk on particular coastal islands off New England, NY, especially during months of May–July when nymphal deer ticks are most abundant; seroprevalence may reach 7% (Shelter Island, NY), but symptomatic cases are uncommon

Pathophys: Intraerythrocytic infection with hemolysis

Incubation period: 7 d to several weeks

Sx: Fever, malaise, myalgias, shortness of breath

Si: Fever, lymphoma-like si (Ann IM 1981;94:327), splenomegaly

Crs: Days–wks of fever; asx carriers, persistent long-term infection unless treated, and subclinical infections all common (Nejm 1998;339:160); may be fatal, esp in elderly, splenectomized, etc.

Cmplc: Acute respiratory failure, DK, CHF, renal failure; r/o ehrlichiosis (16.17), Lyme disease (16.24) or concomitant infection w same

Lab:

Hem: Intra-RBC parasites, look like malaria ring forms; tetrads sometimes seen; PCR has high sensitivity on whole blood (J Clin Microbio 1992;30:2097)

Serol: Indirect immunofluorescence antibody = 1/64 or greater (JID 1994;169:923); hamster innoculation is a definitive test for *B. microti* when smears are negative

Rx:

- Quinine 650 mg or 8 mg/kg tid po + clindamycin 600 mg or 10 mg/kg po (or iv) tid × 7 d (Ann IM 1982;96:601) but tinnitus and abdominal distress result in 20% failing to complete crs (Nejm 1998;339:160)
- Atovaquone + azithromycin, which has fewer side effects (J Trop Med Hyg 1996;55:219; Nejm 2000;343:1454), is equally effective
- Exchange transfusion cures acute hemolytic crisis (Nejm 1980;303:1098)

Prevent: Insect repellants, timely tick removal, etc.

18.8 BLASTOCYSTIS HOMINIS

Guerrant Trop Inf Dis 1999;ch 67:699

Cause: *B. hominis*, an anaerobic protozoan; common GI tract commensal; no clear evidence that it is a pathogen, but controversy persists, and incr prevalence in stools associated w unsanitary conditions

Epidem: Worldwide, but more prevalent in tropics; approx 1% of U.S. residents carry in stool

Risk for travelers: Commonly reported in stool exams of trekkers in Nepal, others w residence in tropics, often w/o assoc w diarrhea

Pathogen: Unknown

Incubation period: Unknown

Sx: usually none; some reports have assoc high #s of organisms in stool w nausea, vomiting, abdominal pain, diarrhea

Si: None

Rx: In vitro sensitivity to metronidazole, Tm/S, furazolidone; benefits of rx unproven

18.9 CHAGAS' DISEASE (AMERICAN TRYPANOSOMIASIS)

Nejm 1993;329:639; 1991;325:763

Cause: *Trypanosoma cruzi*

Epidem: Endemic from U.S.–Mexico border to southern So America (see Fig. 18.2); most U.S. cases occur in immigrants from endemic areas; prevalence rates up to 5% in high-risk immigrants from endemic areas (Am J Med 1987;82:915); transmitted by reduviid beetle ("kissing bug," "barbeiros") at night, usually in habitations with adobe wall, thatch etc., which provide insect niche; trypanosome stage in blood ingested by reduviid (triatoma) insect, multiply in insect's GI tract into metacyclic stage; bug infected for life, no vertical transmission; metacyclic stage in feces near bite, enters wound or transferred manually by host to eye and elsewhere; multiplication only in intracellular form, which then ruptures, leading to trypanosomes in blood

Animal (rodent) reservoirs: Central and So America; rarely via blood transfusion (Ann IM 1989;111:849, 851) or congenital if placental defect

Risk in travelers: Very rare (Exposure dependent on sleep in infested dwellings)

Incubation period: Acute sx, incl chagoma, or unilat periorbial swelling (Romãna's si) in 1–2 wk; chronic sx over yr; acute form in children; chronic in adults who had acute form in past

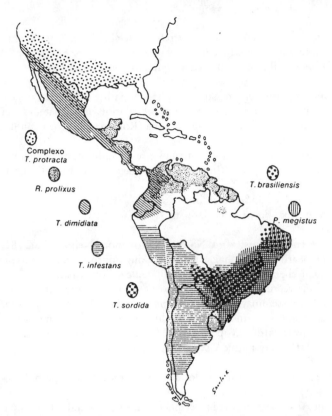

Figure 18.2. Geographic distribution of the most important species of triatomids transmitting *T. cruzi*. (Reproduced with permission from Tropical Geog Med.)

Pathophys:

Acute form: infection of muscle fibers, glial cells, and others; after rupture, fibrosis and granulomas develop

Chronic form: autoimmune reaction leads to cardiac fibrosis; diminished ganglionic cells in gut leads to esophageal and colon dilatation

Sx:

Acute: fever, facial or lower extremity swelling, small persistent nodule from bite (usually on face)

Chronic: CHF, GI sx of megaesophagus and megacolon

Si:

Acute: hepatosplenomegaly, lymphadenopathy; chagomas = local tissue swelling in skin at site of inoculation of parasite, especially in children; unilateral eye swelling (Romaña's si) with conjunctival involvement

Chronic: CHF (especially ventricular heart failure), heart block, angina, Vtach, or other cardiac involvement in 30–40% eventually

Crs:

Acute: 4–6 wk, 5% mortality

Chronic: sx appear years later in 10–30%

Cmplc:

Acute: encephalitis, asx CNS disease common (Nejm 1978;298:604); myocarditis, r/o Chagas whenever any appropriately exposed pt has ischemic heart disease or dilated cardiomyopathy

Chronic: recrudescence w immunosuppression can reactivate with HIV, dissemination with transplant (CID 1998;26:177), different geographic strains assoc with different complc, ie some with chagasic cardiomyopathy, others with megadisease; presentation in AIDS may mimic CNS toxo w mass lesions

Lab:

Bact: *Acute*: culture from blood or tissue on NNN (type of blood agar)

Hem: *Acute*: organisms in peripheral smear, especially buffy coat; prominent kinetoplast; undulating membrane. *Chronic*: no organisms

PCR based assays may have utility

Noninv: Thallium ETTs and EKGs appear like MI, RBBB, R ventrc enlargement common (Circ 1987;75:1140)

Path: *Chronic*: organisms in tissue sections in only 25%

Serol: *Acute*: comp-fix titer elevated but hemagglutination titer increased first; *Chronic*: IgG ELISA titer (sens/specif as yet unspecified); or comp-fix titer (Ann IM 1969;71:983) all have a high false-pos rate; radioimmune precip assay more specific

Rx: None very good

Acute: nifurtimox (Rev Infect Dis 1986;8:884) 8–10 mg/kg/d po divided qid × 120 d; alternative, benzimidazole

Chronic: combination of itraconazole/allopurinol may have some
   utility (Am J Trop Med 1998;59:133)
Prevent: Vector control through proper housing construction; for
   travelers who must sleep in poorly constructed dwellings (ie, in
   village adobe hut structures, etc. in endemic areas), consider bed
   nets, use of insecticide on walls, etc.

18.10 CLONORCHIASIS, LIVER FLUKE

Nejm 1984;310:298
Cause: *Clonorchis sinensis, Opisthorchis* sp
Epidem: E and SE Asia, including Taiwan; embryonated egg in feces is
   ingested by snail where becomes a miracidium, then a sporocyst,
   and eventually redia (2nd site of multiplication); then evolve to
   free-swimming cercaria, which penetrate under fish scales and are
   ingested, mature into adults, which migrate to bile ducts; animal
   reservoirs, dogs and cats; common wherever poorly cooked fish
   eaten, especially in the Far East
Risk in travelers: Rare, but a prevalent infx in many parts of Asia
Incubation period: wk–yr
Pathophys: Adults survive 30⁺ years causing fibrosing response
Sx: Light to moderate infx is asympt; heavy can cause various GI sx
   (Lancet 1996;347:194); note that an acute syndrome w fever,
   abd pain, eosinophilia can occur
Si: Mild hepatitis, RUQ abd tenderness, hepatomegaly
Crs: Chronic (yrs) infx
Cmplc: Recurrent ascending cholangitis; cholangiocarcinoma (rare)
Lab: Eosinophilia common
   Bact: Stool smear shows embryonated eggs, also in duodenal
      aspirates
   Serol: Capture ELISA (monoclonal Abs) has 70% sensitivity
   Xray: Characteristic abd echo, CT findings: cystic or mulberry-like
      dilatations; moving linear echoes on ultrasound
Rx: Praziquantel 25 mg/kg tid × 2 d (Ann IM 1989;110:290) or
   albendazole
Prevent: Avoid undercooked fish

18.11 CRYPTOSPORIDIUM DIARRHEA (AND OTHER COCCIDIA—CYCLOSPORA, ISOSPORA, ETC.)

Nejm 1994;331:161; 1985;312:1278; Ann IM 1996;124:424

Cause: *Cryptosporidium parvum*

Epidem: Worldwide; fecal–oral dissemination from humans or cattle (Am J Pub Hlth 1989;79:1528) or contaminated water supplies (Nejm 1994;331:161), even those w filtered water treatment systems (Ann IM 1996;124:459)

Risk for travelers: Common cause of prolonged traveler's diarrhea; person-to-person household spread is common in tropics (Ann IM 1994;126); may infect up to 50% of AIDS pts in Haiti, Africa

Pathophys: Oocysts excyst w/i lumen of small bowel; release sporozoites, which enter microvillous border; eventual cell invasion by merozoites

Incubation period: 1 wk (average)

Sx: Usually watery, nonbloody diarrhea (86–93%) × 12 d average; occasional abdominal cramps (84%); vomiting (48%); anorexia (20%); fever (12–57%); weight loss (20%); nausea (12%)

Si: Usually none

Crs: 6–22 d course; all recover in immunocompetent host (Nejm 1986;315:1643); cause of voluminous diarrhea (3 L/d) and wasting syndrome in AIDS patients

Cmplc: Chronic cholecystitis/cholangitis as well as dissemination in AIDS and other immunocompromised patients; r/o similar intestinal spore-forming protozoa (Ann IM 1996;124:429): *Cyclospora cayetanensis*, coccidia-like organism, larger than cryptosporidia (Nejm 1993;328:1308); causes fatigue and malabsorption w chronic infection (Ann IM 1995;123:409; 1993;119:377) in travelers and waterborne epidemics (Central American imported raspberries; Nejm 1997;336:1548) and especially in AIDS pts; prophylaxis and rx w Tm/S is effective (Ann IM 1994;121:654); *Enterocytozoon bienensis*, intracellular microsporidial protozoan (Nejm 1992;326:161); causes diarrhea and cholangitis (Nejm 1993;328:95; Ann IM 1993;119:895); *Isospora belli*, common in tropics, where it is a major cause of chronic diarrhea in pts with AIDS; can cause persistent diarrhea (wk–mo) in some travelers; rx with Tm/S or pyrimethamine (Ann

IM 1988;109:474; Nejm 1986;315:87); sarcocystosis; common in rural Asia, but found throughout tropics; usually w/o sx, but may cause intestinal disease, along w muscle encystation; may cause necrotizing eosinophilic enteritis

Lab:

Bact: Ziehl–Neelsen acid-fast stain of stool for O + P; 10% false neg; 75% still have present in stool after sx subside (Nejm 1986;315:1643); ELISA-based detection tests show promise (J Clin Micro 2001;39:332)

Rx (cryptosporidiosis): Supportive; and, if necessary, as in AIDS, paromomycin 500 mg po tid × 2 wk, 500 mg bid maintenance; spiramycin, azithromycin, or furazolidone have been used, but with little success

Prevent: *Cryptosporidia* are chlorine-resistant; public water systems need excellent filtration/treatment; for travelers, wash fruits/vegetables, drink iodine treated or boiled water or use small pore filters; pts w AIDS need to be particularly careful

18.12 CYCLOSPORA

Guerrant et al; Trop Inf Dis 1999; ch 69; CID 2000;31:1040

Cause: *Cyclospora cayatenensis*

Epidem: Tropics; cases mostly occur during summer or rainy season

Risk for travelers: Common cause of traveler's diarrhea in trekkers in Nepal, other areas; during rainy season, 7% of U.S. embassy personnel acquired infx (Lancet 1993;341:1175)

Incubation period: 2–14 d

Sx: Watery diarrhea, cramps, weight loss

Si: Usually none

Crse: Can last wk (7 d–6 wk); severe diarrhea may occur in pts w AIDS

Lab: Positive stool smear on modified acid fast; larger than *Cryptosporidia* (8–10 microns)

Rx: Tm/S, one DS qd × 7 d (Lancet 1995;345:691)

18.13 CYSTICERCOSIS (LARVAL PORK TAPEWORM INFECTION)

Ann Rev Med 2000;51:187

Cause: larval *T. solium* (human is intermediate host)

Epidem: Worldwide; high prevalence in Latin America, Asia, SubSaharan Africa; prevalence in Latin America 20%; leading cause of adult onset seizures in Mexico City; acquired by ingestion of tapeworm eggs shed by a carrier, usually via contaminated food or water; transmission in household in U.S. documented from employed carrier (Nejm 1992;327:692)

Pathophys: Ingested eggs give rise to oncospheres that penetrate stomach, enter circulation, and lodge in CNS (predominantly), but also in retina, heart, subcutaneous tissue, muscle; cysts develop, clicit minimal inflammatory rxn; can persist 2–10 or more yr; when cyst degeneration begins, antigens leak out, causing intense inflammatory rxn

Risk in travelers: Rare

Incubation period: Yrs

Sx: Usually seizures, also can cause headache (chronic meningitis, inc ICP), mental status changes, visual sx

Si: May have focal neuro changes

Lab/Xray: Brain CT or MRI (preferred)—findings depend on cyst stage; early—small contrast enhancing lesions, often at gray matter–white matter junctions; ring enhancement with degeneration; scolex may be identified; after degeneration, small calcific nodules remain

   Serol: Modified immunoblot using parasite glycoproteins (enzyme-linked immunotransfer blot—CDC) has excellent sensitivity (except for solitary lesions) and specificity

Rx: Symptomatic for seizure; antiparasitic treatment controversial, but usually favored except if very limited parenchymal disease or old calcific lesions (Arch IM 1995;155:1982); praziquantel (50–100 mg/kg/d dosed tid for 2 wk) or albendazole (15 mg/kg/d in divided doses × 28 d); dexamethasone may be added for severe inflammatory rxn w rx

Prevent: Avoid potentially ova-contaminated foods (ie, fresh salads, vegetables) in highly endemic countries (ie, Mexico, Central and

So America, etc.); heating food over 60°C or freezing kills ova; cysticerci in pork also killed by freezing (Jama 1986;256:893)

18.14 ECHINOCOCCAL (HYDATID) CYST DISEASE

Cause: *Echinococcus granulosus* (cystic hydatid disease), *E. multilocularis* (alveolar hydatid disease), *E. vogeli* (polycystic hydatid disease)

Epidem: Rural areas (eg, sheepherding) in temperate zones, Middle East and No Africa (*E. granulosus*); arctic and alpine foci in Europe (*E. multilocularis*), No So America and Panama (*E. vogeli*); see Fig. 18.3; most U.S. cases are in immigrants, esp Iranian, Iraqi, Syrian (Am J Trop Med Hyg 1995;53:668); humans are only intermediate host, ie, do not spread eggs in stool; transmitted fo humans by ingestion of encysted organisms from fecal–oral contamination of dog/other animal feces

Risk in travelers: Rare (no data); most US cases in immigrants from endemic areas

Incubation period: Yrs

Pathophys: Like a neoplasm, echinococcal cysts grow over years with appearance of secondary cysts

Sx: Variable, depending on location, size of cysts; majority are in liver, less frequently lung (*E. granulosus*)

Si: Mass effects anywhere; hepatomegaly, jaundice

Crs: Cysts develop over yrs

Lab:
  Serol: for *E. granulosus*—ELISA, IHA titers increased (from CDC) are pos in 90% with liver, 75% with lung involvement; for *E. multilocularis*, use ELISA or immunoblot with specific antigens; false-positive reactions are common

  Xray: Ultrasound + CT reveal cysts; internal septae due to daughter cysts may be seen

Rx: Albendazole 5 mg/kg po tid × 28–56 d + either surgical or percutaneous drainage (Nejm 1997;337:881)

Prevent: Avoid fecal–oral exposure to conaminated soil, etc.

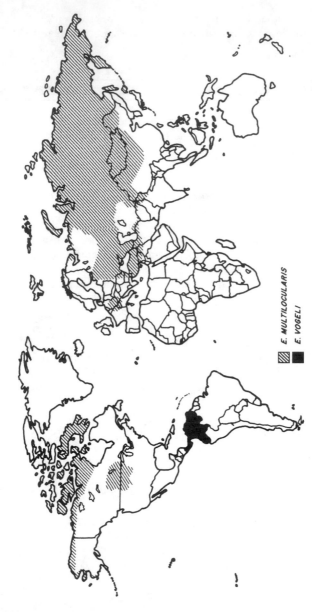

Figure 18.3. Geographic distribution of *E. multilocularis* and *E. vogeli* infections. (Reproduced with permission from Tropical Geog Med.)

18.15 ENTEROBIASIS (PINWORMS)

Cause: *Enterobius vermicularis*
Epidem: Worldwide; female lives in colon and lays eggs in perianal region; there reinfected to same host or others by scratching; no tissue penetration; 30% of U.S. population under age 20 gets it, all social classes
Risk for travelers: Mostly peridomestic rather than travel related; more common in temperate than in tropical areas
Pathophys: Rarely invasive
Sx: Anal pruritus, vaginitis
Si: Perianal excoriation (uncommon)
Crs: Chronic infestation common w/o Rx
Cmplc: Vaginitis can lead to migration into peritoneal cavity where granulomas form; rarely appendicitis
Lab:
  Bact: Scotch tape to perianal area early in AM, then paste on slide to examine under microscope to see characteristic eggs, flat on one side (sensitivity 50% 1 swab, 90% w 3)
Rx: Mebendazole (Vermox) 100 mg × 1, repeat in 2 wk (Nejm 1977;297:1437); or pyrantel 11 mg/kg (1 g max) × 1, repeat in 2 wk; or albendazole; rx all family members at same time, even if asx since probably all have

18.16 FASCIOLIASIS AND PARAGONIMIASIS

Guerrant et al, Trop Inf Disease 1999; ch 100
Cause:
  Fascioliasis: *Fasciola hepatica* (sheep liver fluke), *fasciola gigantica*
  Paragonimiasis: *Paragonimus westermani*, others
Epidem: Similar to clonorchis except metacercaria encysts on water plants (fascioliasis) or crustaceans (paragonimiasis)
  Fascioliasis: worldwide wherever sheep raised and human manure used to fertilize salad foods (watercress, etc.); 2 million infected worldwide (esp Bolivia, Peru, Iran, Egypt, Portugal)
  Paragonimiasis: mink farms in U.S.; Southeast Asia, W So America (uncooked or pickled crabs, crawfish, shrimp)

Risk for travelers: Rare–very rare (no data)

Incubation period:

Fascioliasis: 6–12 wk

Paragonimiasis: acute sx 2–15 ds; may present wk to yr later

Pathophys:

Fascioliasis: in adult, "snowplows" through liver to reach biliary system

Paragonimiasis: hypersensitivity response to encysted adults

Sx:

Fascioliasis: acute (2–4 mo) fever, urticaria, RUQ abd pain, nausea; chronic–intermittent biliary obstruction

Paragonimiasis: diarrhea, abd pain followed by cough, urticaria, hemoptysis, pleurisy, seizures (brain cysts)

Si: Fascioliasis: fever, hepatosplenomegaly

Crs:

Fascioliasis: chronic infx may persist for 3–5 yrs

Paragonimiasis: 5–10 yrs

Cmplc:

Fascioliasis: intermittent biliary obstruction, cholangitis

Paragonimiasis: pleuropulmonary disease, rare CNS disease

Lab:

Bact: stool, sputum, urine show operculated eggs (paragonimiasis); yield increased with concentration; AFB of Gram's stain may interfere with detection on sputum; (*Fasciola*) typical eggs in stool, duodenal aspirates

Hem: eosinophilia (sometimes)

Serol: (fascioliasis) ELISA capture antigen test; (paragonimiasis) CF tests (CDC), ELISA, antigen detection

Xray: Chest xray with paragonimiasis may resemble tbc (variable but can include nodules, cavities, diffuse infiltrates); ultrasound (fascioliasis): multiple hypodense lesions, esp branching funnel-like peripheral lesions; CT scan (paragonimiasis) shows grape-like clusters of cysts; fascioliasis: abd CT may show hypodense liver lesions w tracks

Rx:

Fascioliasis: Bithionol (Nejm 1972;287:995) (adverse effects: pneumonias as organisms killed); triclabendazole also effective, well tolerated (CID 2001;33:1)

Paragonimiasis: Praziquantel 25 mg/kg tid × 1 d (Ann IM 1989;110:290)

Prevent: Do not eat undercooked crustaceans, or unwashed salad foods

18.17 FILARIASIS (OVERVIEW)

Cause: *Wuchereria bancrofti* (elephantiasis), *Onchocerca volvulus* (blinding worm—Nejm 1978;298:379; see 18.19), *Loa loa* (eye worm; see 18.18), *Brugia malayi* (elephantiasis), *Dirofilaria* sp (dog filariasis), and perhaps tropical eosinophilia (TE) is also a form of filariasis from an unknown worm (TE; Nejm 1978;298:1129); *Mansonella* sp may cause skin lesions w/o systmic sx

Epidem: Tropics and subtropics; all transmitted by flies or mosquitoes (*Brugia* and *Wuchereria*); take a long time to mature, hence up to a yr for onset of sx; 2-week maturation in insect; infect via puncture holes; males and females in lymphatics produce microfilarial worms, which migrate to peripheral blood in diurnal fashion where ingested by insect and thus complete cycle

Lymphatic filariasis; tropics; onchocerciasis limited to parts of Africa/Central and So America; *Loa loa* is limited to rainforest areas of W Africa (see Fig. 18.4) in tropical areas; *Dirofilaria* occasionally in U.S.

Risk for travelers: Rare; occasional cases in long-term travelers, Peace Corps volunteers, etc.; however, worm burden is low, and therefore sx usually limited to hypersensitivy rxn to parasite

Pathophys: Adults block lymphatics, fibrotic nodules form about them in lymphatics or in sc locations (*Onchocerca* and *Loa*); TE probably is an infection w worms whose microfilaria never get into blood; are in nodes and lung biopsies; nonimmunes get hypersensitivity rxn; antigen-specific suppressor cells produced cause filaremia (Nejm 1982;307:144); recent recognition of presence of co-factor bacteria (*Wolbachia*), which is an endosymbiont of filaria (Lancet 2001;357:1415)

Incubation period: Several months to years after exposure

Sx: Onset may be delayed up to 5$^+$ yr after leave area; skin rashes, esp w oncho; local swelling and redness of skin where microfilaria enter (migratory angioedema); fever, Calabar swelling (*Loa*): a swelling of 2–3 cm sc anywhere but often in areas of trauma; subconjunctival movement of worm ("eyeworm") sometimes noted; lymphatic fialariasis: filarial fevers w painful adenopathy followed by retrograde lymphangitis (adenolymphangitis)

Si: Recurrent lymphangitis especially of extremities, male genitalia; can see worms crawling sc often (*Loa*) especially in loose sc tissue, eg,

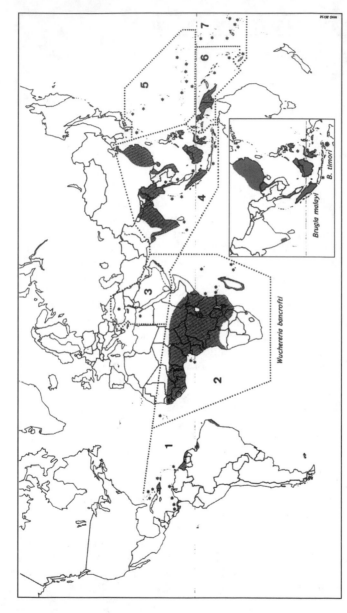

Figure 18.4. Distribution of lymphatic filariasis and vector zones. (Reproduced with permission from WHO, *Lymphatic filariasis*, WHO Technical Report Series 702, 1984.)

eye, scrotum, breast, penis; Calabar swellings w *Loa*; chronic
rash w oncho; in chronically infected pts, lymphedema
(lower extremities, scrotum)

Crs: Chronic sx w high worm burden, but self-limited in most travelers

Cmplc: Blindness (*Onchocerca*) w chronic exposure; lymphatic
obstruction (chronic); but in expatriates picture is more often
recurrent angioedema, rash, eosinophilia

Lab:

Hem: eosinophilia; microfilaria in blood sporadically (not in TE or
Onchocerca), 40% pos thin smears; thick smear better, or spin
crit and look at buffy coat smear under low power; yield may
be increased by concentration (Knott technique); time of day
important for different species (ie, *Loa* circulates 4 PM local time);
provocative test (Mazzoti): rx w DEC × 1; draw blood 15 min
later and examine for microfilaria

Urine: hematuria, proteinuria may be present w *W. bancrofti*

Path: biopsy of lymphatics or skin nodules (*Loa, Onchocerca*) show
adults; in oncho, skin snips w PCR or microscopy is diagnostic

Serol: Positive for filaria-specific IGG, but not species specific; rapid
card test now available

Rx: Single dose ivermectin (120 mg/kg) = DEC (6 mg/kg/d in 3 div
doses for 2–3 wk) for lymphatic filariasis (Nejm 1990;322:1113);
DEC preferred for Loa loa; albendazole may have role (adulticidal
and microfilariacidal)

Prevent: Use of insect repellants, bed nets, vector control;
diethylcarbamazine 300 mg po q 1 wk prevents *Loa loa*
(Nejm 1988;319:752)

18.18 FILARIASIS: LOAIASIS

Guerrant Trop Inf Dis 1999; ch 80:861

Cause: *Loa loa*, a filarial nematode

Epidem: Coastal plains (especially rainforest) of W and central Africa
(see Fig. 18.5); vector is red tabanid fly

Risk for travelers: Low; occasional cases in expatriates, long-term
travelers/visitors who stay several mo or more in endemic areas

Pathophys: Immunologic rxn to worm antigens

Incubation period: months to yrs

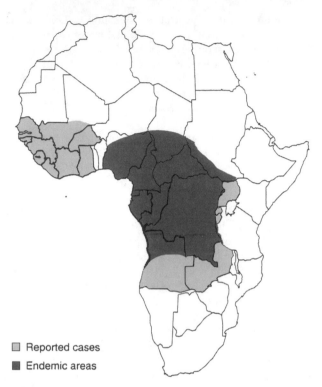

☐ Reported cases
■ Endemic areas

Figure 18.5. Distribution of *Loa loa*. (Reproduced with permission from Tropical Infectious Diseases.)

Sx: Transient migratory swellings (Calabar swellings), esp on face, extremities; recurrent urticaria; conjunctivitis (occasional siting of subconjunctival "eyeworm"; these sx often more pronounced in nonresidents (ie, nonimmunes)

Si: Angioedematous (nonpitting) swellings w/o erythema; occas sc nodules

Crs: Recurrent sx over mos to yrs

Compl: Renal disease; encephalitis (sometimes triggered by rx of filaria)

Lab: Extraction of adult worm; detection of microfilaria in daytime blood (but rare in nonimmunes to find mf); high grade eosinophilia usually present

Serol: IgG 4 antigen w high sensitvity, but not specific for filarial species

Rx: DEC (see doses above) kills mf, maybe adults; be aware it can trigger systemic hypersensitivity rxn; surgical removal of adult worm may be helpful if possible

Prevent: Insect repellants, etc.; also weekly DEC has been employed (see above)

18.19 FILARIASIS: ONCHOCERCIASIS

Lancet 1998;351:1341

Cause: *Onchocerca volvulus*, a filarial nematode

Epidem: Equatorial Africa; small foci in Central, So America (Mexico, Guatemala, Ecuador, Guyana); see Fig. 18.6; vector is blackfly (*Simulium* sp); habitat is rapidly flowing rivers and surroundings

Risk for travelers: Rare; disease usually requires repeated exposures over mos to yrs; recent recognition of infx in shorter term "adventure travelers" (BMJ 1992;304:1285)

Pathophys: Inflammatory rxn to larval/adult worms in skin, eye (corneal scarring, uveitis)

Incubation period: 1–2 yr; worms live in host 5–10 yrs

Sx: Pruritus (often intractable), eventual lichenification of skin; conjunctivitis; localized sc nodules

Si: Diffuse papular eruption, sc nodules (0.5–3 cm) often over bony prominences, sacrum

Cmplc: Chronic pruritic rash; blindness ("river blindness")

Lab: Skin snip of nodule w PCR (JID 1994;169:686) or microscopy (use corneoscleral bx to obtain it; bx of nodule also revealing)

  Serol: Rapid format antibody card available for antibody detection in field (JID 2000;182:1796)

Rx: Ivermectin (120–150 m/kg single dose); Nejm 1985;393:133); may require repeat Rx q 6 mo for 5–10 yr

Prevent: Insect repellants, vector control (major international effort underway); possible new strategy w mass Rx of population w ivermectin, followed by doxycycline to eradicate microfilaria (Lancet 2001;357:1415)

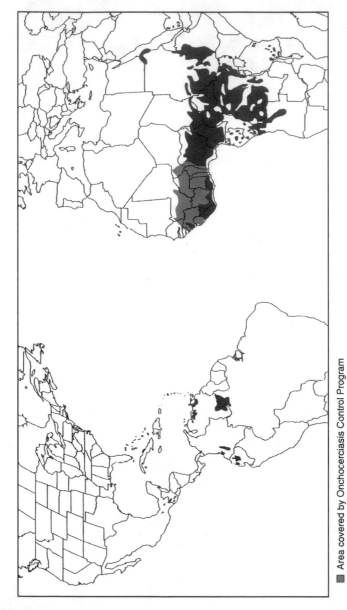

Figure 18.6. Distribution of endemic *onchocerciasis*. (Reproduced with permission from Tropical Infectious Diseases.)

■ Area covered by Onchocerciasis Control Program

18.20 GIARDIASIS

Nejm 1978;298:319; CID 1997;25:545

Cause: *Giardia lamblia*

Epidem: Worldwide; epidemic (food and water borne) and sporadic transmission; peak incidence in late summer in U.S., UK, Mexico; encysted form excreted in feces, ingested by new host, resides in duodenum; animal reservoirs: beaver, dog, muskrat, perhaps deer

Occurs in areas of poor sanitation with raw rural surface (not ground) water; day care settings; associated with globulin deficiencies, especially of IgA; achlorhydria, nodular lymphoid hyperplasia

Risk for travelers: Common cause of traveler's diarrhea in Russia; common in campers, hikers and can be transmitted by swimming in contaminated water; also common in Peace Corps volunteers in tropics (J Clin Micro 2001;39:34)

Pathophys: Malabsorption due to mechanical obstruction of duodenum by covering microcilli

Incubation period: 1–3 wk

Sx: Loose, watery stools (93%), malaise (80%), bloating and cramps (75%), fatigue, weight loss (73%); true diarrhea in only 30%; Ddx incl cryptosporidiosis, cyclosporiasis; traveler's diarrhea, which often does not start until return from a trip, ie, delayed onset

Si: Usually none

Crs: Can persist for wks

Cmplc: Malabsorption; rare extraintestinal sx (urticaria, reactive arthritis); lactose intolerance develops in 20–40%

Lab:

Bact: Stool O + P, 70% false neg; 2 "eyed" (nuclei) flagellated trophozoite, or 4 nucleated cyst; 3 stools 70–90% sensitive; string test (Enterotest) samples duodenum w high sens, but cumbersome

Serol: Giardia antigen in stool (sens 85–98%, spec 90–100%)

Rx: Active disease:

- Metronidazole (Flagyl), 1st, 250 mg or 5 mg/kg tid × 5–7 d; or alternatively
- Furazolidone 100 mg or 1.25 mg/kg qid × 5 d; no carcinogenicity
- Tinidazole (not available in U.S.)

- In 1st trimester of pregnancy, consider paromomycin
  (25–30 mg/kg/d × 7 d)

Prevent: Avoiding sewage contamination of water supplies; filtration; iodine as 2% solution, 0.4 cc/L of water; or heating to 70°C (158° F) × 10 min (Am J Pub Hlth 1989;79:1633); chlorination probably inadequate even at 8 mg Cl⁻/L × 10 min; backpackers/campers can prevent w appropriate filters (<1 micron)

18.21 GNATHOSTOMIASIS

Guerrant Trop Inf Dis 1999; ch 87:941

Cause: *Gnathostoma* sp

Epidem: Common in Thailand, Japan; sporadic cases elsewhere; acquired by ingestion (or handling) of raw or undercooked freshwater fish and amphibians; third-stage larvae in fish penetrate stomach and "wander" in host

Risk for travelers: Rare, but high attack rates have been reported in small outbreaks; one involved 8 of 12 diplomats in Bangladesh who ate raw fish pate (Wilson ;1991:517); occasionally dx in Asian immigrants; recent incr in cases from Mexico

Incubation period: Few days to yrs; GI sx usually soon; soft tissue swelling 3–4 wk

Sx: Epigastric pain, nausea, vomiting for 1–3 wk; then may get migratory soft tissue swellings, serpiginous skin rash

Si: Migratory soft tissue swellings; cutaneous larva migrans rash; urticaria; rare neuro si

Crs: Mild to severe; soft tissue swelling may be red, last few wk, resolve and reappear elsewhere over mo; migratory larvae may inv nervous system (enccphalitis) or eye

Lab: Usually eosinophila; dx based on path of worm

Rx: Supportive

Prevent: Avoid raw/undercooked fish

18.22 HOOKWORM

Nejm 1984;310:298; Guerrant et al, Trop Inf Dis 1999, ch 91

Cause: *Ancylostoma duodenale* and *Necator americanus*

Epidem: Worldwide; larvae penetrate skin in filariform stage (5 d older than rhabditiform stage), or larvae ingested in feces; Africa, So America, Far East, southern Europe, U.S., especially in south with barefoot children and poor sewage; nearly 200 million in China estimated infected

Risk for travelers: Rare–very rare (no data); symptomatic infx requires large worm burden

Incubation period: For "ground itch," days

Pathophys: Skin penetration, into circulation, thence to lung, into trachea, to pharynx where swallowed and then attach to small intestine, where they result in chronic blood loss

Sx: Papulovesicular dermatitis may occur for 1–2 wk; w large worm burden, fatigue

Si: Anemia, 150–200 cc/d with *Ancylostoma* when severe infestations; *Necator* 1/5 as much, ~0.03 cc/d/worm

Crs: Adult hookworms can persist 1–9 yr in bowel

Cmplc: CHF; r/o *Ancylostoma caninum*, dog hookworm, which can infect humans and cause abdominal pain, eosinophilic gastroenteritis, partic common in Australia (Ann IM 1994;120:369)

Lab:

Bact: Stool O + P shows eggs same size as ascaris, w thin delicate shell; hatch in 24 h into rhabidiform larvae, which molt into filariform larvae; can quantify eggs and estimate number of worms

Hem: Hgb as low as 1–3 g; Fe deficiency anemia

Rx:

- Mebendazole (Vermox) 100 mg bid × 3 d; or albendazole (400 mg single dose); neither ok in pregnancy; alt rx—pyrantel pamoate
- $FeSO_4$ for the anemia

Prevent: Mass geohelminth rx in populations; improved sanitation

18.23 LARVA MIGRANS/TOXOCARIASIS (CUTANEOUS AND VISCERAL)

Nejm 1985;313:986; Ann IM 1994;120:369

Cause:

Cutaneous, "creeping eruption": Ancylostoma braziliense and *caninum*

Visceral: Toxocara canis, T. cati, raccoon ascaris and others

Epidem:

Cutaneous: common in tropical/subtropical areas; many cases in U.S./Canadian travelers to beach resorts of Caribbean, Mexico (Arch Dermatol 1993;129:588); from contact with soil; dog and cat hookworm larvae penetrate skin but never get into circulation; children get when crawl under buildings

Visceral: worldwide; ingestion of dog feces w eggs; 20% of U.S. dogs have it; eggs survive several winters; 10% of adults in U.S. have serologic evidence of it

Risk for travelers: *Cutaneous*: low to moderate for in particular Mexican/Caribb beach resorts; VLM very rare (pediatric)

Incubation period: *Cutaneous*: 2 wk (range 1–120 d)

Pathophys:

Cutaneous: larvae in skin cause local inflammation; cannot penetrate dermal/epidermal junction

Visceral: worms invade viscera, where permanent granulomas form

Sx:

Cutaneous: raised serpiginous itchy areas of skin advance up to 1–2 cm/d (creeping eruption); mean # of lesions = 3, often on lower extrem (CID 1994;19:1062)

Visceral: age 1–4 yr usually; often asx or erratic fever, anorexia, rash, seizures, wheezing, cough

Si:

Cutaneous: rash

Visceral: hepatosplenomegaly, tumor-like growths in eye in older children (ocular VLM) have been mistaken for retinoblastomas

Crs:

Cutaneous: self-limited, × several wk (may develop impetigo, allergic rxns)

Visceral: self-limited

Cmplc: *Visceral*: eosinophilic meningoencephalitis (Nejm 1985;312:1619)

Lab:

Hem: Eosinophilia in both types; hypergammaglobulinemia

Path: *Visceral*: bx (usually not justified since benign crs) of liver, lungs, CNS, muscle show eosinophilic granulomas

Serol: *Visceral*: ELISA titer for *T. canis* = 1/32 (78% sens, 92% spec) get kit from CDC

Stool: No eggs in either type

Rx:

Cutaneous: albendazole (400 mg single dose; cure rate 50–100%; CID 2000;30:811) or ivermectin (12 mg po single dose; cure rate 70–100% w 1–2 supplemental doses; CID 2000;31:493)

Visceral: diethylcarbamazine 2 mg/kg tid × 7–10 d; or albendazole (10 mg/kg/d × 5 d); or mebendazole; steroids for eye disease

Prevent: Avoid direct skin contact w sands, soils contam w dog, cat feces

18.24 LEISHMANIA: VISCERAL (KALA-AZAR) AND MUCOSAL/CUTANEOUS

Nejm 1993;328:1383; Ann IM 1993;118:779 (cutaneous); 1990;113:934

Cause: *Leishmania donovani* (kala-azar); *L. tropica*, *L. major*, and *L. braziliensis* (mucocutaneous), others

Epidem: Scattered foci on all continents except Australia, Antarctica, but most prevalent in tropics (see Figs. 18.7A and 18.7B); approx 30–40 cases cutaneous and several visceral cases treated in U.S. travelers per year, esp adventure travelers or field biologists, and in immigrants; arthropod-borne transmission; sandfly ingests parasitized cell, ruptures, and becomes leptomonad stage, which reproduces in fly gut, then migrates to mouth parts where is injected with next bite and, as leptomonad stage, migrates to RES cells where becomes leishmania form, which burst and invade other cells

Vectors sandfly genera *Lutzomyia* (Americas) and *Phlebotomus* (Eurasia, Africa); animal reservoirs (eg, dogs, rodents, sloths); human-to-human contact transmission also possible, skin-to-skin

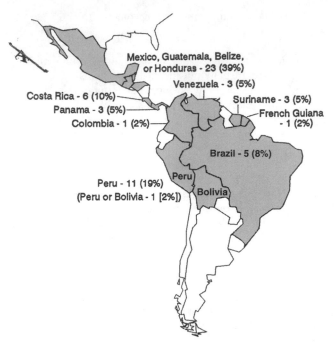

Figure 18.7A. Countries in which study patients (n = 59) acquired American cutaneous *leishmaniasis*. (Reproduced with permission from Annals of Internal Medicine 1993;118:781.)

in cutaneous types; indigenous in Asia, Africa, Middle East, and tropical So America, where there are 2000 cases/2 million/yr

Pathophys: Organisms in macrophages; suppressor T cells keep delayed hypersensitivity to leishmania antigens turned off (Nejm 1982;306:387); cutaneous lesions often heal only to develop mucocutaneous disease years later

Risk for travelers: Low; as noted above, most cases in U.S. seen in immigrants; some cases in biologists, ecotourists, military in jungle training (17 soldiers out of 500 infected during jungle training in Panama; Wilson, 1991)

Incubation period: Cutaneous/mucocutaneous: few wks–several mos; visceral; 2–8 mos

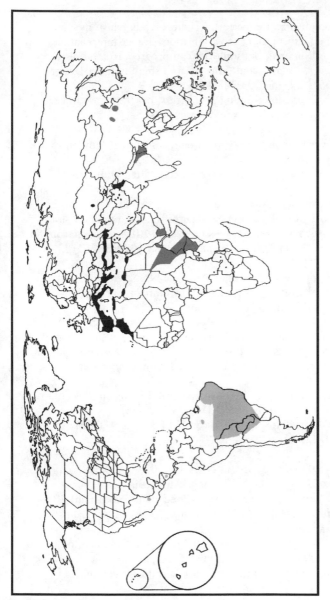

Visceral Leishmaniasis
  Leishmania (L.) chagasi
  Leishmania (L.) donovani
  Leishmania (L.) infantum

Figure 18.7B. Distribution of visceral leishmaniasis. (Reproduced with permission from Tropical Infectious Diseases.)

PARASITIC DISEASE

Sx:

Kala-azar: long incubation period, weight loss, diarrhea; in some cases, hyperpigmentation; most infections are asymptomatic or mild and self-limited, but minority can progress to fatal disease; chronic fever, malaise, and GI sx seen in small number Desert Storm troops (Nejm 1993;328:1383)

Mucosal/cutaneous: slow-healing skin ulcers, nasal mucosa, other areas of oropharynx in severe disease

Si:

Kala-azar: fever (intermittent or remittent, sometimes daily biphasic), hepatosplenomegaly

Mucosal/cutaneous: chronic (mos–yrs) ulcers, often with raised borders, scars

Crs: *Kala-azar*: chronic, fatal without rx

Cmplc: *Kala-azar*: GI and pulmonary superinfections; rarely amyloid and cirrhosis; many reports of kala-azar in AIDS patients from So Europe, some with aplastic anemia (J Infect 1990;21:261)

Lab:

Bact: Culture all above on special media (ie NNN, etc.)

Hem: Depressed white counts, anemia, thrombocytopenia, hypogammaglobulinemia (kala-azar)

Path: Typical, 1–3 μ *Leishmania*–Donovan bodies (amastigotes) in monocytes, lymph nodes, spleen, skin lesions, marrow, liver; distinguish from histo by kinetoplast; for cutaneous form, punch bx split for culture, touch prep (stained with Wright's or Giemsa) and histopath

Serol: ELISA, IFA, others; often negative in HIV; Recomb nk 39 sens/spec for visceral disease (JID 1996;173:758)

Rx: Consult CDC at 404-639-3670 (see Med Lett Drugs Ther 1998;40:1–12)

1st:

- Allopurinol 20 mg/kg qd in qid doses × 15 d, eg, 300 mg po qid (Nejm 1992;326:741); no help w mucocutaneous form
- pentavalent antimony as sodium stibogluconate (Pentostam) 20 mg Sb/kg/d iv/im × 21–28 d (toxicity includes pancreatitis, cardiac) or meglumine antimoniate
- α interferon 100 μgm/m^2 im qd × 10 d results in 90% cure of cutaneous and visceral (Nejm 1990;322:16); but not yet clearly 1st choice (Nejm 1990;322:55); 70% cure in mild–moderate

mucocutaneous type but only 20% in severe disease (Ann IM 1990;113:934)
- For Indian visceral leishmaniasis, miltefosine (Nejm 1999;341:1795)
  Alternatives: amphotericin B, or pentamidine
Prevent: Use of DEET-containing insect repellants and permethrin treated clothing is helpful when in endemic areas, also use fine mesh bed netting at night (CID 1996;22:1), population-based measures have included residual DDT use and reservoir animal control

18.25 MALARIA

Clin Inf Dis 1998;27:142; Guerrant Trop Inf Dis 1999;ch 70:736
Cause: *Plasmodium vivax, ovale, malariae, falciparum*
Epidem: Worldwide; 200–300 million cases/yr (WHO); resurgent in many areas due to failure of mosquito control efforts, resistance of mosquito to insecticides (incl residual DDT), and resistance to commonly used antimalarial treatments; risk is seasonal in many regions

Distribution: *vivax* in Southeast Asia, So America; *ovale* in W Africa; *malariae* is found worldwide, but most prevalent in Africa; *falciparum* is common in Africa, Oceania; also SE Asia, So America, India and some areas of Caribbean (ie, Haiti)

Vector: anopheles mosquito; patients heterozygous for Hgb S, C, E, or G6PD may be more resistant; Duffy blood group FyFy completely protected vs *vivax* (Nejm 1976;295:302); transmission may also be congenital or by blood transfusion

Pathophys: 3–4 h fevers, as endotoxins, including tumor necrosis factor (Nejm 1990;320:1586), are released when schizonts rupture into merozoites synchronously in blood. *Vivax* infects young (retics) RBCs only; *malariae*, old RBCs only. *Falciparum* infects all RBCs and causes "sticky" RBCs, which infarct brain, kidney, lung (Nejm 1968;279:732); no exoerythrocytic phase, hence no late recurrences; *vivax* and *ovale* forms may reside in liver, reemerge as primary or secondary hypnozoites wks to mos later

Risk to travelers: See malaria prevention (Chapter 4); geographic risk varies in unprotected tourists substantially from 1–2%/mo in W Africa to 0.01%/mo in So America; but attack rates may be much higher locally, and w frequent exposure to vector mosquitos; MOST COMMON CAUSE OF FEVER IN TRAVELERS SEEKING EVALUATION ON RETURN FROM TROPICS; ALWAYS CONSIDER MALARIA UNTIL PROVEN OTHERWISE

Incubation period: Average 2 wks; most *P. falciparum* presents w/i 1–2 mo; *P. vivax* (esp temperate strains) may range to 9–12 mo; 50% *vivax* present w/i 2 mo; in semi-immunes it may be longer

Sx: All malarias may present w backache, myalgias, nausea, vomiting, abd pain, dry cough; fever occurs in paroxysms w rigors; sweating stage follows 2–6 hr later

Vivax: 6–15 d incubation, tertian (qod) fever but 2 crops can cause qd fevers

Malariae: 20–25 d incubation, quartan (q 3 d) fevers

Ovale: tertian fevers

Falciparum: fevers variable at onset; NOTE that *falciparum* may present w prominent GI/resp sx; irregular fever, confusion, ha, etc; eventual development of tertian pattern may be after days of hectic fevers

Si: Splenomegaly (*vivax* = 25%, *falciparum* = 80%); black water fever is hemoglobinuria from massive hemolysis (*falciparum*) possibly triggered by quinine Rx

Crs: 3.5% mortality for *falciparum* in children, usually within 24 hr, especially if change in consciousness, jaundice, respiratory distress, or hypoglycemia (Nejm 1995;332:1399)

Cmplc:

Vivax: tropical splenomegaly syndrome (Nejm 1984;310:337)

Malariae: recurrence decades later possible (Nejm 1998;338:367)

Falcip: DIC (Ann IM 1969;70:134); CVA, coma (steroids no help; Nejm 1982;306:313); hypoglycemia correlates with severe *falciparum* disease and diminished hepatic gluconeogenesis, associated with severe morbidity and mortality in 50% (Nejm 1988;319:1040); see Table 18.1

r/o babesiosis in U.S. (see 18.7)

Lab:

1. Microscopy is gold standard (Am J Trop Med Hyg 2000;63:76); check thick/thin smear (Giemsa preferred); if initial smear neg, check × 3 over 6–12 hr; sensitivity is 80–90% for *P. falciparum* in experienced labs; thick smears are important to dx low parasitemias; thin smears provide better definition for species

Table 18.1. Criteria for severe malaria (P. falciparum)

Asexual forms of P. falciparum on blood smear
AND
Any one or more of the following:

Coma or any sign of cerebral dysfunction
Severe normocytic anemia
Pulmonary edema
Hypoglycemia
Hypotension
Spontaneous bleeding (with DIC or thrombocytopenia <20,000)
Renal failure
Repeated generalized seizures
Acidemia/acidosis
Jaundice
Parasitemia 4% (nonimmunes)

Adapted from World Health Organization (2000) Severe falciparum malaria. Transactions of the Royal Society of Tropical Medicine and Hygiene 94: supplement 1.

PARASITIC DISEASE

identity; NOTE: ASSUME *P. FALCIPARUM* UNTIL PROVEN OTHERWISE; if parasites easy to find, have lab determine level of parasitemia (# asex parasites /oil immersion field; examine 10–20; or % parasites/1000 RBCs on thin smear)

Hem: vivax, single infections of only young (big) RBCs; circulating older ameboid trophozoites and schizonts; 16 merozoites/schizont; Schüffner's dots (small, eosinophilic) in RBC; *ovale*, oval RBC often fringed at one end; *ovale* and *malariae*, "band-like" trophs; 8 merozoites/schizont; *falciparum*, multiple infections of each RBC; all ages and sizes of RBCs; only young, small ring trophozoites (older trophs and schizonts in RES); 24 merozoites/schizont; Mauer's dots in RBC (eosinophilic, larger)

2. Nonmicroscopic dx methods: immunologic: antigen capture— immunochromatographic methods (parasight F kit; PATH; ICT) have 90+% sens/spec for *P. falciparum*; ICT, OPTIMAL assays (Am J Trop Med Hyg 2000;63:76; 2000;63:139) have high sens for *vivax*; some false pos w some assays may occur w + rheumatoid factor PCR: sensitivity comparable to microscopy thick smear (CID 1998;27:142); DNA probes: less sens than PCR, but nearly comparable to thick smear; antibody detection: detectable after 8–10 d of infx; useful in retrospect/epidem studies

3. Other lab: thrombocytopenia (60–80%); WBC nl or low (90%); inc LDH (70–80%)

Rx: (Nejm 1996;335:800) (CDC phone number: **770-488-7788**);
Also: (WHO) Trans Roy Soc Trop Med Hyg 2000;94;suppl1:1

Treatment strategy; if species undx, treat for *P. falciparum*; assume chloroquine resistant unless only exposure was in the few areas of chloroquine sensitivity; determine parasitemia if *P. falciparum*, admit, and determine po vs iv fluids; if parasitemia >5% or severe malaria, start w iv rx

For all malarias EXCEPT choroquine resistant *P. falciparum*:
- Chloroquine 600 mg base (1 g), then 300 mg at 12, 24, and 36 hr; or in severely ill, 10 mg base/kg iv over 8 hr then 15 mg/kg over 24 hr, or 35 mg/kg im/sc q 6 hr or via NG + for prevention of relapse in vivax/ovale malaria add:
- Primaquine phosphate 26.3 mg/d (15 mg base) × 14 d or 79 mg/wk 945 mg base) or q week for 8 wks; check G6PD status first; for prevention of relapse in *vivax* malaria acquired in SE Asia, Somalia, where resistance to primaquine may occur, consider double dose (Am J Trop Med Hyg 1995;52:322); note: chloroquine resistant *P. vivax* may occur in India, Iran, Papua New Guinea, So America; treatment failures can be treated w regimens noted below plus primaquine

Resistant *falciparum* (CRPF) (adult dosage):
- Quinine sulfate 650 mg po tid × 3–7 d, with
- Tetracycline 250 mg qid (or doxycycline 100 mg bid × 7 d) **OR**
- Clindamycin 900 mg po tid × 3 d, **OR**
- Follow quinine rx w 3 tabs pyrimethamine/sulfadoxine (Fansidar) single dose on last day

Alternatives to these regimens incl (adult dosage):
- Mefloquine 750 mg po followed by 500 mg po 12 hr later, or
- Malarone 2 (adult dose) tabs bid × 3 d (w food)

If iv rx needed: monitor w ECG
- Quinidine gluconate 10 salt mg/kg over 1–2 hr iv, then 0.02 salt mg/kg/min constant infusion until can take po + exchange transfusion if >10% RBCs infected (Nejm 1989;321:65)

Alternative Rx: Cerebral and severe *falciparum* malaria:
- Quinine 10 mg/kg iv/im q 8 hr after 20 mg/kg initial dose, over 4 hr w 5% dextrose, or
- Artemether 2 mg/kg im q 8 hr after 4 mg/kg load (Nejm 1996;335:69, 76, 124)

- Deferoxamine iron chelation speeds recovery *in falciparum* pediatric cerebral malaria by denying organism its vitamins! (Nejm 1992;327:1473)

Patients from border areas of Thailand w possible multi-resistant *P. falciparum*:
- Consider malarone or combination rx w artemisin plus mefloquine.
- Check w CDC for detailed advice as rx approaches for this area rapidly change

Prevent: See Chapter 4 on malaria prevention and chemoprophylaxis

---

18.26 SCHISTOSOMIASIS

Nejm 1984;310:298; 1980;303:203; Ann IM 1982;97:740

Cause: *Schistosoma mansoni, japonicum,* and *haematobium;* less common *S. mekongi, intercalatum;* swimmers itch from *S. dermatidis*

Epidem: Tropics (see Fig. 18.8), including Africa, Asia (including Indonesia, Phillipines), So America, parts of the Caribbean; 200 million infected worldwide; assoc with cutaneous exposure to freshwater (usually slow running streams, lakes, etc.); free-swimming cercaria penetrate skin or ingested, become schistosomula in blood and mature into adults in blood vessels; they then deposit in body tissues selectively (*S. mansoni* and *S. japonicum* about GI tract, *S. haematobium* about bladder); they mate and lay eggs that work out to feces or urine, are excreted into water, where become miracidium, which invades a snail and reproduces again, and eventually are released as cercaria; can live 30–40 yr in humans

In *S. dermatidis* swimmer's itch, only cercarial penetration of skin by nonhuman schistosomes occurs; cycle stopped there

S. mansoni in Caribbean, Africa, Middle East; *S. haematobium* in Africa, Far and Middle East; *S. japonicum* in Far East (Nejm 1983;309:1533); *S. dermatidis* in marine or fresh water

Risk for travelers: Rare, but outbreaks w high attack rates reported in adventure travelers (Omo River rafters, etc.), students swimming in infested lakes or streams (Lancet 1996;348:1274; Mmwr 1993;42:565); asymptomatic infx may occur in up to 18% of travelers to endemic areas w fresh water exposure

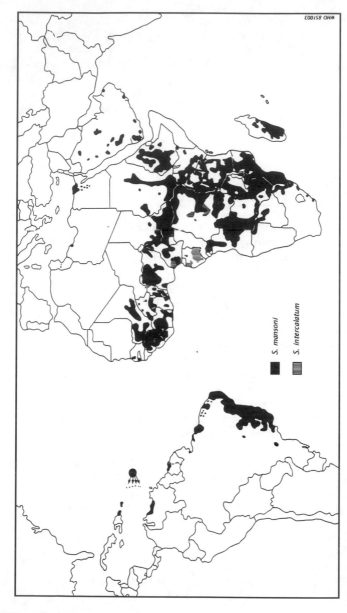

Figure 18.8. Distribution of schistosomiasis due to *Schistosoma mansoni* and *S. intercalatum*. (Reproduced with permission from WHO, *The Control of Schistosomiasis*, WHO Technical Report Series 728, 1985.)

S. mansoni

S. intercalatum

Incubation period: Cercarial dermatitis (skin rxn to exposure) w/in 24 hr; acute febrile illness (Katayama fever) in nonimmune persons 4–8 wk postexposure; other sx mos to yrs

Pathophys: Focal granulomas, fibrosis, vasculitis, or hypersensitivity rxn (acute disease in nonimmune pt); swimmer's itch due to allergic reaction to worms on 2nd exposure.

Sx: Chills, diarrhea, abdominal pain, weight loss, bloody urine/stool; acute (4–8 wks postinfection) hypersensitivity form (Katayama fever), fever, headache, cough, pruritus (Jama 1990;263:2165); also acute transverse myelitis in nonimmune travelers; recent reports of primarily respiratory sx/si in some travelers w acute schistosomiasis (Am J Med 2000;109:718)

S. dermatidis: swimmer's itch

Si: Hepatosplenomegaly (70%), fever (60%), diarrhea (60%); in acute hypersensitivity, fever, urticaria, lymphadenopathy, hepatosplenomegaly

S. dermatidis: skin welts or swelling

Crs: Adult worms produce eggs over 4–7 yr

Cmplc: Granulomatous response to eggs anywhere including brain, skin, liver with cirrhosis and varices, GU tract with obstruction and secondary infections (Ann IM 1971;75:49) and immune complex nephritis (Ann IM 1975;83:148)

Swimmer's itch: r/o sea bather's eruptions from anemone medusae (Nejm 1993;329:542)

Lab:

Bact: stool/urine show typical eggs: *S. japonicum*, round; *S. haematobium*, single-tailed; *S. mansoni*, forked-tailed; can visuallize with direct smear or concentration methods

Hem: eosinophils increased

Serol: FAST ELISA plus Western blot more sensitive/specific (Clin Lab Med 1991;11:1029) when obtained several mos after infx; urine dipstick has sensitivity of 50%

Rx: Treat symptomatic pts and seropositive travelers (Trans Roy Soc Trop Med Hyg 2000;531)

- Praziquantel 20 mg/kg bid × 1 d; good vs all types; 70–85% cure (Nejm 1984;310:298); metrifonate (*S. haematobium* only) or oxaminoquine (*S. mansoni* only); seroids for acute hypersensitivity reactions
- Swimmer's itch, no rx

PARASITIC DISEASE

Prevent: Avoid freshwater contact (ie, swimming, wading) in endemic
   areas; towel off immediately if exposure occurs; water left
   standing for 48–72 hr is safe for use for washing, etc., as is
   chlorinated water or water heated to 122°F

18.27 STRONGYLOIDES INFECTIONS

Arch IM 1987;147:1257; CID 1996;23:949

Cause: *Strongyloides stercoralis*

Epidem: Worldwide, esp tropical, humid areas; skin penetration by
   filariform, migrates to blood vessels, thence to lung, from there up
   to the pharynx, where is ingested back down the GI tract where
   imbeds and produces live young, which are released into feces;
   can mature in GI tract and autoreinfect or mature on the ground;
   increased prevalence in institutions for retarded; southern areas

Risk for travelers: Low (little data); high prevalence in some military
   personnel living in poor conditions during WWII and Vietnam
   war, some immigrant populations (esp refugee); dissem disease
   assoc w HTLV 1

Incubation period: Wks to yrs

Pathophys: Usually minimal GI damage; in hyperinfection, much tissue
   damage in GI tract; perhaps exotoxin release; as noted above, may
   in severe cases develop internal autoreinfection

Sx: Abdominal pain, midepigastric; nausea, vomiting and diarrhea;
   perineal pruritus

Si: Urticaria, larva currens rash (migratory dermatitis)

Crs: May persist >30 yr in active stage

Cmplc: Hyperinfection with dissemination may occur in
   immunosuppressed pts w colitis, pneumonitis, meningitis
   Superinfections w secondary gram-neg bacteremias, bowel obstruction
   and malabsorption in pts w diminished resistance, eg, on steroids
   (can cause death if already infected; Nejm 1966;275:1093),
   Hodgkin's, leukemia, SLE, leprosy (Ann IM 1970;72:199)
   Acute pneumonitis due to sensitivity reaction w tissue migration

Lab:
   Bact: stool shows rhabditiform larvae in feces sporadically; must use fresh stool, neg in 25%–50% w single exam; duodenal aspirate best and most reliable

   Hem: eosinophilia (50%)

Rx:
- Ivermectin (200 μg/kg for 1–2 d; JID 1994;169:1076) effective and well-tolerated
- Thiabendazole 25 mg/kg (3 g max) bid × 2 d; both tissue and intestinal phases hit; cure in 65%; side effects in 50%

Prevent: Wear shoes, dig latrines

18.28 TAPEWORMS

Nejm 1992;327:692, 696, 727; 1984;310:298

Cause: *Taenia saginata* (beef), *T. solium* (pork); *Diphyllobothrium latum* (fish); *Hymenolepsis nana* (dwarf tapeworm), *Hymenolepsis diminuta*, *Dipylidium caninum* (dog tapeworm)

Epidem: Worldwide, but esp tropics (*T. saginata*, *solium*, *H. nana*); adult worms in "definitive" carnivore hosts (dog, bears, etc.), eggs in feces eaten by humans or herbivorous animal ("intermediate hosts") and then encyst in muscle, etc.; in *T. solium* and dwarf tapeworm, humans can be a definitive host or an intermediate host (muscle encystment) via autoinoculation or fecal–oral transmission, eg, in food handlers or in families; humans are only definitive hosts, ie, worm is in GI tract

   Seen especially in children and the retarded; dwarf tapeworm is most common in U.S.; *T. solium* is endemic in Mexico, central America and in many immigrants, eg, in California, where CNS clinical presentation my be due larval stage (cysticercosis)

Risk in travelers: Low–rare (no data risk assoc directly with eating habits re: undercooked meat, etc.)

Incubation period: Days to weeks

Pathophys: Bowel commensals

Sx: *Taenia* and *D. latum*: rarely cause sx (abdom pain, nausea) beside complaints of passage in stool; dwarf: diarrhea and occasionally obstructive GI sx

Si: None

Crs: Adult tapeworms can live 25 yr

Cmplc: *D. latum*: B_{12} and folate deficiencies; *T. solium* larval disease from ingestion of eggs: cysticercosis in brain, muscle, and skin (50%); sx may take 4–5 yr to develop when larva dies (Nejm 1984;311:1492)

Lab:

Bact: stool O + P shows characteristic ova and gravid segments (except in cysticercosis)

Serol: IHA titers increased with *T. solium* cysticercosis

Rx: Adult forms, in GI tract, of *Taenia*, *D. latum*, and dwarf:

- Praziquantel 5–10 mg/kg × 1; 99% effective (Ann IM 1989;110:290); others recommend 10–20 mg/kg (Med Lett 1998;40:1) or
- Niclosamide 2 g (500 mg under age 2, 1 g age 2–12 yr) once (89% cure), then 1 g (500 mg age 2–12 yr) po qd × 5 d

T. solium cysticercosis: surgical excision; albendazole (15 mg/kg/d divided doses × 28 d; Arch Neurol 1995;52:104) or praziquantel + dexamethasone (Nejm 1984;311:1492; Ann IM 1983;99:179)

Prevent: Adequate cooking or freezing of beef, pork, fish; (pickling in brine, salting are unreliable)

18.29 TOXOPLASMOSIS

Nejm 1985;313:957; 1978;298:550; Ann IM 1976;84:193

Cause: *Toxoplasma gondii*

Epidem: Worldwide; many animal reservoirs; cats are primary hosts, usually transmitted via cat feces? contaminated water (Nejm 1982;307:666) or dust (Nejm 1979;300:695); also from poorly cooked meat; 15–30% of U.S. population have had; especially in wet hot areas; immunosuppression can induce; fetus very susceptible; 40% contract disease when mother gets primary infection between 2–6 mo gestation (Nejm 1974;290:110); increased in AIDS as an opportunistic infection

Risk for travelers: Low, though prevalence higher in warmer climates than in U.S.

Pathophys: Inflammation and scarring in brain, liver, spleen, heart, eye; cysts are inert; eye lesions probably are due to delayed

hypersensitivity reactions; congenital form somewhat different
clinical pattern than acquired

Incubation period: 1–3 wk

Sx:

Acquired (Nejm 1979;300:695) (90%): fever, headache (85%),
myalgia (60%), rash (20%)

Congenital: rash

Si:

Acquired: lymphadenopathy (85%), rash (20%), chorioretinitis

Congenital: chorioretinitis (100%), icterus, rash, hepatosplenomegaly,
hydrops, hydrocephalus

Crs: Parasites may persist in host for life

Cmplc: Acquired: meningoencephalitis (50%), r/o lymphoma
(Ann IM 1969;70:514); myocarditis

Lab:

CSF: congenital: organisms on Wright's stain and grow in mice

Path: intracellular blue with red cytoplasm; can look like intracellular
"grapes" when multiplying in cell; do brain bx in AIDS patients
w meningoencephalitis if do not respond to pyrimethamine +
clindamycin within 2 wk (Nejm 1993;329:995)

Serol: indirect fluorescent antibody positive if >1:1000; comp-fix
antibody and Sabin–Feldman dye test (interpretation of various
mother/child combinations; Nejm 1978;298:550); IgM titers now
available

Xray:

Acquired: CT of head shows focal encephalitis with enhancing rings
(Nejm 1988;318:1439)

Congenital: in utero, cerebral calcifications and bony "white puffs"

Rx:

Congenital: prevent w screening titer at 1st ob visit, then q 1 mo toxo
titers (if elevated but stable, no problem), and in exposed seroneg
pregnant women; abort if convert and fetal infection documented,
eg, by amniocentesis PCR methods (Nejm 1994;331:695); or
rx with spiramycin; or pyrimethamine + sulfa, which results
in 13/15 healthy newborns, other 2 had only retinitis (F-Nejm
1988;318:271); or screen newborns for IgM toxo titers; this
detects 1 case/6000 infants in New England and subsequent rx
allows prevention of future eye disease (Njem 1994;330:1858)

Acquired: 1st choice pyrimethamine 25–100 mg/d or 2 mg/kg/d × 3 d
then 1 mg/kg/d up to 25 mg + sulfadiazine 1–2 g or 25–50 mg/kg

qid × 3–4 wk; or pyrimethamine + clindamycin 1200 mg qid
(Nejm 1993;329:995; Ann IM 1992;116:33), which is preferable
in AIDS because 40% of such pts cannot tolerate sulfa; alternative
is spiramycin 3–4 g/kg or 50–100 mg/kg/d × 3–4 wk

Eye involvement: steroids

Prevent: Care w handling uncooked meat; cooking kills parasite; care w
handling of cat feces—dispose of in <24 hrs to minimize risk

18.30 TRICHINOSIS

Jama 1983;249:23; Nejm 1978;298:1178

Cause: *Trichinella spiralis*, 4 other species

Epidem: Worldwide; highest incidence in Asia, So America, Mexico;
T. nativa common in arctic (JID 1989;160:513)

Life cycle: infection on ingestion of meat w cysts, hatch and
reproduce for 6 wk in GI mucosa, living young born and many
get into skeletal muscle, where grow and encyst, some calcify, and
others remain viable for years; from pigs fed uncooked garbage;
polar and other bears

Risk in travelers: Very rare

Incubation period: Acute GI sx w/in 72 hr of ingestion, but 7–30 d is
typical for disease presentation

Pathophys: Invasion of skeletal (not heart) muscle by worms,
degeneration of invaded fiber causing inflammatory reaction,
and finally, encysted larvae (in all other tissues this reaction
kills larvae)

Sx: Fever, myalgias all over including tongue, diaphragm, etc.;
gastroenteritis 24–72 hr after ingestion from worms in GI tract;
in arctic form, GI sx predominate

Si: Eye swelling (50%), conjunctivitis, small conjunctival hemorrhages;
splinter hemorrhages in nail beds; skin rashes both urticarial and
petechial

Crs: GI sx in 24–72 hr; other sx peak 1–6 wk after ingestion; may
persist for wks in arctic form

Cmplc: Myocarditis, CNS inflammation

Lab:

Chem: CPK, AST (SGOT) markedly elevated in 50%

Hem: elevated eosinophils; may be as high as 50%

Path: muscle bx shows 10–100 larvae/g tissue; = 1/g should not produce sx

Serol: After 3 wk infx, use ELISA IGG (most sensitive), indirect IFA, or charcoal flocculation test; crossreact in autoimmune diseases; recommend use of 2 different tests to increase specificity

Rx: disease (Med Let 1998;40:1):

- Mebendazole 200–400 mg po tid × 3 d, then 400–500 mg po tid × 10 d or albendazole
- ASA for mild disease or
- Steroids to decrease inflammation if becomes life-threatening but they also increase life of adult worms

Prevent: Cook garbage fed to pigs; cook or freeze pork well (−15°C × 20 d); note that *T. nativa* is resistant to freezing

19 Arthropod Bites and Infections

19.1 LICE

CID 1999;29:888

Cause: *Phthirus pubis* (crabs; Nejm 1968;278:950); *Pediculus humanus* (body lice); *P. capitis* (head lice)

Epidem: *P. pubis*, venereal; *P. humanus* and *P. capitis*, via bedding, clothing, and other fomites

    Life cycle: 25 d egg-to-egg; live exclusively on human blood, cannot live >24 h without it; only ~10 adults/pt. Body lice are vectors for relapsing fever (Ethiopia), trench fever (Bartonella quintana), and epidemic typhus.

Pathophys: Attach to hair; itch and rashes due to bites and allergies to louse and its feces

Sx: Pruritus with all; *P. pubis* localized to axillary, perianal, pubic areas, and occasionally in eyelashes (blepharitis)

Si: Lice and nits (egg sacks on hairs) evident w magnifying glass or careful inspection; bites

Cmplc: r/o bird lice (eg, from pigeons on air conditioner)

Rx: (Med Let 1997;38:6)

    Launder clothes, bedding; hang them outside × 24 h will also kill since cannot survive >24 h away from body

    Meds: rx as below and repeat × 1 at 7d (? resistant lice controversial; Lancet 2000;356:524)

    • 1st: permethrin 1% (Nix); $9/2 oz; 95% cure with 1 rx at 14 d (Am J Pub Hlth 1988;78:978)

    • 2nd:

      1. Permethrin 5% (Elimite) over night, or

      2. Lindane shampoos (1% gamma benzene hexachloride, Kwell), × 1 usually enough; may need × 3 q 4 d; $5/2 oz, or

3. Pyrethrins + piperonyl butoxide (Rid, Vonce, A-200, Pronto); 65% cure after 1 rx at 14 d (Am J Pub Hlth 1988;78:978); $5/2 oz
* 3rd: Ivermectin (Mectizan) 200 µgm/kg po × 1

Rx of eye cmplc, 1/4% eserine ophthalmic ointment to lids with cotton tip applicator; of school outbreaks, full guidelines; "nit free policies unrealistic"

19.2 MYIASIS

Arch Dermatol 1990;126:199

Cause: Larvae (maggot) of (botfly) *Dermatobium hominis* fly, African tumbu fly, others

Epidem: Human botflies common in forested areas from Mexico to So America; tumbu flies in tropical Africa

Risk for travelers: Low, but cases regularly seen in ecotourists, adventure travelers, etc. returning from tropics of Central/So America.

Pathophys: Egg introduced by fly or on mosquito into skin; matures over several wk into sizeable maggot w subcutan swelling; sometimes secondary infx

Sx: Pain, itching, sense of "movement" in boil under skin

Si: Furuncular lesion(s) w central aperture

Dx: Posterior spiracles of larvae can often be visualized in aperture; dx also made after excision

Rx: Extraction of larva, sometimes difficult due to horizontal alignment in lesion; lidocaine sc into lesion anesthetizes larva and patient; may be brought to surface w occlusion of aperture (esp w tumbu fly); see fascinating report on use of bacon rx for botflies (Jama 1993;270:2087)

Prevent: Appropriate clothing to deter mosquitos/flies, use of insect repellants (note botfly larvae can penetrate clothing)

19.3 SCABIES: COMMON AND NORWEGIAN

Ann IM 1983;98:498; Nejm 1978;298:496; 1968;278:1099

Cause: *Sarcoptes scabiei* var. *hominis*: an arthropod mite

Epidem: Norwegian rare in U.S. except in AIDS pts and alcoholics; contagious w close contact

Risk for travelers: High prevalence in developing countries; close contact w infested individuals or their bedding/clothing

Pathophys:

Common: burrows in skin, leading to allergic reaction

Norwegian: no burrowing, but hides beneath skin scales

Sx:

Common: itching, worst at night

Norwegian: no itching

Si:

Common: red papules in intertriginous areas

Norwegian: hyperkeratotic skin hiding mites

Crs:

Common: even w rx takes 2 wk for sx to subside

Lab:

Bact: Mineral oil scraping of burrow shows mite or eggs under low power

Rx: (Med Let 1993;35:111)

Launder clothes, bedding; hang them outside × 24 h will also kill since cannot survive >24 h away from body

Meds:

- 1st, permethrin 5% (Elimite) cream × 8–12 h; 30 g enough to rx adult; 91% cure; safer than lindane
- 2nd, lindane 1% (Kwell) once though often may need repeat; 86% cure; crotamiton 10% (Eurax) if above fails; 60% cure
- Experimental: ivermectin 200 μg/kg po × 1, very effective, esp w crusting type and/or in immunosuppressed (Nejm 1995;333:26)

19.4 TICK PARALYSIS

CID 1999;29:1435

Cause: Neurotoxins inroduced by a biting (attached) tick; can occur w bites of female ticks of 40 species; usually assoc w *Dermacentor* sp in U.S. (ie, dog or wood ticks)

Epidem: Worldwide; most cases reported from No America, and Australia; most often dx in children

Risk for travelers: Rare

Pathophys: Specifics unknown; illness reversible w tick removal

Incubation period: 4–5 d post-tick attachment (so ticks that cause this are usually in hair or other hard to inspect area)

Sx: Starts w irritability, paresthesias (1–2 d); then ascending weakness over hr to d

Si: Bilat flaccid paralysis Ddx: Guillain–Barré syndrome, botulism

Crs: Dep upon finding tick; up to 10% mortality reported if dx not made

Rx: Dramatic response to removal of tick

Prevent: Tick repellants; "tick checks" on children

19.5 TUNGIASIS

Wilson, 1991: 680

Cause: *Tunga penentrans*, the chigoe flea or jigger (not the chigger mite); infests swine, other animals

Epidem: Tropics, esp Africa, C and So America; also Indian subcontinent; larvae live in sandy soil, can jump 35 cm

Risk for travelers: Common in some areas among the shoeless (barefoot) traveler

Incubation period: Minor irritation at time of bite; significant sx 8–12 d later as flea enlarges to size of small pea

Pathophys: Local irritation by presence of enlarging insect under skin

Sx: Pain, itch at sites of bites

Si: Black dot at center of papule = posterior end of female flea; usually in toe webs, under nails, or on ankles

Crs: Persistent sx for 1 mo until flea disgorges eggs and deflates; residual itch persists in some

Rx: Remove w scalpel blade or sterile needle and forceps

Prevent: Cover feet; avoid direct contact of skin w soil

20 Viral Infections

20.1 ALPHAVIRUSES

Guerrant Trop Inf Dis 1999;Ch 119;1281

Cause: Mosquito-borne RNA viruses; chikungunya in E and W Africa, India, SE Asia; Barmah Forest virus in Australia; Ross River in Australia and So Pacific; Mayaro in So America and Trinidad (CID 1999;28;67); Sindbis virus (Old World—all continents); endemic in these areas w sporadic outbreaks

Risk for travelers: High attack rates may occur w all residents; during epidemics; in Australia, Ross River causes >1000 cases in some yr (Wilson, 1991); incubation period 2–10 d (range from 2–21)

Pathogen: Different viruses have different tissue tropisms (ie, Ross River and joints)

Sx: Acute onset fever (often biphasic in chikungunya); arthralgias; maculopapular rash; retro-orbital pain; GI sx (nausea, diarrhea) common w Mayaro fever

Si: Fever: symmetrical arthritis (ie, Ross River virus); rash, lymphadenopathy

Crs: Acute illness lasts 5–10 d; chronic sx may develop in Ross River and chikungunya infx w yrs of joint pain (1/4 w joint pain at 1 yr in one study (S African Med J 1982;63:313)

Rx: Supportive

Prevent: Use of mosquito preventive measures

20.2 ARBOVIRAL ENCEPHALITIS

Guerrant Trop Inf Dis, 1999, ch 118; Ann IM 1969;71:681-St. Louis type; CID 1999;28:882 (tick-borne encephalitis, or TBE)

Cause: St. Louis, Eastern equine, Western equine, other arboviruses (U.S.); Venezuelan equine encephalitis (So America); Japanese encephalitis (Asia, Malaysia); tick-borne encephalitis (Central Europe, Russia, China); Murray Valley virus (MVV; Australia); Rift Valley virus (Africa); West Nile virus (WNV) (Africa, Europe, and introduced into U.S. 1999)

Epidem: Geographic/ecological risk varies w type; most are mosquito borne.

St. Louis: urban *Culex* mosquito from birds and invertebrates (Nejm 1967;277:12); incidence up in adults age >40 yr; many unapparent cases

E. equine: mosquitoes and/or ticks from wild birds. In Eastern U.S., incidence up after rainy winter; <100 cases in literature; kills horses by 1000s and children age <10

W. equine: rural *Culex* mosquito, from birds and snake reservoirs; incidence in infants and adults age >50 yr; 3000 cases in 1959; endemic in Columbia River basin; many inapparent cases

TBE: carried by *Ixodes ricinus/I. persulcatus* ticks; associated w Alpine pasture and wooded areas; highest incidence in Latvia and Urals; W. Siberia; occurs across Europe from east Switz to Urals, and from Scandinavia to Italy, but highly focal

Japanese encephalitis: see map (Fig. 3.6) and CDC table (Table 3.7); associated w *Culicine* mosquito, especially in rice farming areas w presence of swine; recent expansion to Nepal, Pakistan, Papua New Guinea; incidence 10–100/100,000 in endemic areas; epidemics occur generally north of Tropic of Cancer, April–Oct, rainy season

Risk for travelers: Rare; particular types of travel may incr risk (ie, hiking in endemic areas of Alps at 1000 m for TBE, extensive nocturnal outdoor exposure to mosquitos in endemic JE areas); note that raw goat's milk may be a vehicle for transmission of TBE in endemic areas; risk of JE very low for short-term travelers (ie, <1/million) but incr w residence in endemic agricultural area during transmission season to 1/5000; incubation period variable; most between 7–28 d

Sx: Fever, severe headache, nausea, and vomiting, sometimes rash; may precede encephalitic sx by a few days; gait abnormality prominent in Murray Valley virus; motor weakness in WNV

Si: As above; vary as to assoc neuro si w type of encephalitis, conjuctival injection, pharyngitis common w JE

St. Louis: impaired mental status (86%); frontal lobe si (78%); stiff neck (71%); cranial nerve palsies, especially of III, IV, VI, VII (22%); Babinski (30%); seizures (10%)

Crs:

- *St. Louis:* 10–21 d; 16% mortality; 66% if seize
- *E. equine:* 36% mortality; 35% of survivors had neurologic morbidity; both predicted by CSF WBC counts and serum hyponatremia (Nejm 1997;336:1867)
- *W. equine:* 10% mortality; 60% neurologic morbidity
- *JE, MVE:* 25% case fatality rate of symptomatic cases; freq neurologic residua; most cases are asymptomatic (for JE, inapparent:apparent disease ratio is 200–300:1); children, elderly at greatest risk
- *TBE:* 0.5–2% fatality of symptomatic cases (residual paresis in 10–40%); 70–90% of cases subclinical
- *WNV:* infrequent mortality in elderly

Cmplc: St. Louis: SIADH in 12% (Ann IM 1969;71:691)

Lab:

Serol:

- St. Louis: hemagglutination and CF
- E. equine: neutralization
- W. equine: hemagglutination and CF titers
- JE: serum, CSF IgM capture ELISA
- TBE: serum, CSF IgM ELISA
- WNV: serum, CSF IgM ELISA

CSF: St. Louis: 98% have >2 WBC; 36% have >100 WBC; protein <100 mg %

Xray: MRI shows basal ganglia and thalamic focal lesions (Nejm 1997;336:1867)

Rx: Supportive

Prevent: Personal protection against arthropod bites w insect repellants, etc.; avoid unpasteurized dairy (TBE); spray to eliminate mosquito population; vaccination available for those at high risk of JE (Nejm 1988;319:641); in Europe, vaccination also available against TBE for those at highest risk

20.3 ARENAVIRUS (NEW WORLD TYPES: HEMORRHAGIC FEVERS)

Guerrant Trop Inf Dis, 1999, ch 111:1191

Cause: Rodent-borne RNA viruses; Junin (Argentine hemorrhagic fever); Machupa (Bolivian hemorrhagic fever; BHF), Guarnarito (VHF); For Old World types, see Lassa Fever (20.13)

Epidem: Highly focal outbreaks in So America related to incr in particular species of rats/other rodents; mechanism of human infx unknown, ? aerosols; often at disturbed areas of forest–field contact; farmers, forest workers at greatest risk, though BHF may be centered in villages

Risk for travelers: Rare, although Peace Corps volunteers, field biologists, etc. are at small theoretical risk; BHF has been spread via person–person by body fluid contact; incr period 6–14 d

Sx: Fever, ha, myalgias, +/– rash; GI/neurologic involvement may follow; then hemorrhagic manifestations in some; no resp sx

Si: Fever, flushing, conjunctival injection, periorbital edema, bleeding gums, purpura, lymphadenopathy

Crs: Up to 20–30% result in severe disease w high fatality w/o rx

Dx: Viral isolation (blood, tissues), ELISA, RT-PCR

Rx: Ribavirin; for Argentine hemorrhagic fever, use of specific immune plasma w/in 8 d is effective

Prevent: Not considered highly contagious, but suspected cases should be put on aerosol as well as universal precautions (CID 2001;32:446)

20.4 BUNYAVIRUS: RIFT VALLEY FEVER, CRIMEAN–CONGO HEMORRHAGIC FEVER, SANDFLY FEVER

Guerrant Trop Inf Dis, 1999, ch 112;1213; Lancet 1993;342:803

Cause: Family of 41 tropical viruses (RNA); 2 can cause hemorrhagic fever syndromes (RVF, CCHF); 3 serotypes for sandfly fever

Epidem:

RVF: W Africa (rainy season), Rift Valley; recent spread to Saudi Arabia (Mmwr 2000;49:9050); mosquito borne

CCHF: tropical Africa; tick borne (*Hyalomma* sp), nosocomial spread common

Sandfly fever: Mediterranean areas, especially Cyprus, Tuscany, Portugal, Spain; June to October when sandflies active

Risk for travelers: Rare; CCHF a risk for campers, hikers in endemic areas; sandfly fever common seasonally in some areas and cases in travelers reported regularly (Scand J Infect Dis 1991;23:451); incubation period 2 d to 2 wk

Sx: RVF: fever, myalgias, ha, retro-orbital pain (same sx for sandfly fever); CCHF: biphasic flu; fever, myalgias, sore throat

Si: Conjunctival injection, fever, sometimes neuro sx, hemorrhagic sx

Crs: RVF usually mild w convalescence 2–3 wk; rare encephalitis, optic neuropathy; CCHF more severe; convalescence may req mos; sandfly fever usually self-limited; rare meningoencephalitis

Lab: Viral culture, ELISA serology tests; for sandfly fever, IFA test

Rx: Ribavirin may be helpful for CCHF

Prevent: Insect/tick bite prevention; isolation in hospital, contact and respiratory (CID 2001;32:446)

20.5 DENGUE

CID 2000;31:144; Guerrant Trop Inf Dis 1999; ch 117:1265

Cause: Flavivirus, 4 serotypes

Epidem: Tropics worldwide; see Fig. 20.1 (50–100 million cases/yr; 500,000 DHF w 25,000 fatalities) incidence incr w recent population incr and urbanization; vector mosquito is *Aedes aegypti* in cities—daytime biter, peridomestic; breeds in debris such as old tires, empty cans, etc.; *A. albopictus* in villages; DHF occurs in children <15 w hx prior infx

Risk for travelers: An increasing risk, esp in Caribbean, Central/So America where there have been recent epidemics; probably under-diagnosed as it is a self-limited illness in travelers (ie, DHF does not occur w/o recurrent infx)

Pathogen: No cross protection between serotypes; DHF results from incr replication in presence of subneutralizing concentration of antibody from prior infection; vasculitis/DIC results; several serotypes circulate in endemic areas

Incubation period: 3–14 d (average 7)

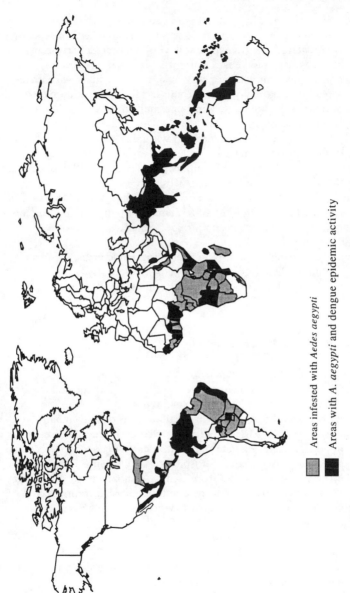

Figure 20.1. World distribution of dengue. (Reproduced from Health Information for International Travel, CDC.)

Areas infested with *Aedes aegypti*

Areas with *A. aegypti* and dengue epidemic activity

VIRAL INFECTIONS

Sx: Acute onset fever, ha, retro-orbital pain, myalgia, nausea; may have sore throat, rash, altered taste sensation; rarely have resp sx or GI sx; in DHF, hemorrhagic sx follow or precede deffervescence

Si: Fever (may have saddleback pattern); conjunctival injection; pharyngitis; lymphadenopathy; rash in 50%; trunk w centrifugal; spread in 2–3 d; may be petechial; facial flushing; desquamation of palms/soles w recovery in some; purpura may develop; rarely encephalitic sx, seizure

Crs: Fever × 5–6 d; convalescence 2–3 wk; DHF has 4 grades of severity w shock, CNS changes in grades 3–4

Lab: Leukopenia, followed by lymphocytosis w atypical lymphocytes; thrombocytopenia; mild incr LFTs

Serology: Send acute/convalescent sera for IgM capture ELISA to CDC Dengue Branch (787-766-5181; email his1@cdc.gov); virus can be isolated in 1st 5 d; sens culture 50%; PCR

Rx: Supportive

Prevent: Habitat modification in endemic/epidemic areas; travelers should use DEET-containing repellants; note *Aedes* mosquitos most active in early AM or late afternoon

20.6 EBOLA VIRUS

Guerrant Trop Inf Dis, 1999, ch 115:1240

Cause: Filamentous RNA viruses that are highly pathogenic for primates, humans; Ebola has 4 subtypes

Epidem: Ebola outbreaks occur in rural areas (forest–savannah interface) of W Africa; epidemics of several hundred cases reported in Sudan, Zaire, Uganda in recent yrs, often assoc w nosocomial spread due to inadequate hospital resources; only a few cases of Marburg virus reported from Kenya, Zimbabwe, So Africa; largest outbreak occurred in Europe due to lab spread from infected Ugandan monkeys; natural reservoirs for these viruses are unknown

Risk for travelers: Remote; few cases reported

Incubation period: 3–20 d

Sx: Acute onset fever, myalgia, pharayngitis, ha, nausea, vomiting; then hemorrhagic sx begin in several days

Si: Fever, maculopapular rash, conjunctivitis, exudative pharyngitis, hemorrhagic si (bleeding from mucous membranes), shock

Crs: 50–90% mortality for Ebola, 20–40% for Marburg

Lab: Antigen capture ELISA is sens/spec; RT-PCR also available; viral isolation is most sensitive

Rx: Supportive

Prevent: Use of sterile needles, barrier isolation (contact/respiratory) precautions in medical facilities when cases suspected (CID 2001;32:946)

20.7 HEPATITIS A (INFECTIOUS HEPATITIS)

Nejm 1997;336:196

Cause: Hepatitis A virus, a pico-RNA enterovirus

Epidem: Worldwide (see map in Fig. 3.3), but incidence rates much higher in many developing countries; fecal/oral contact with infected persons for up to a year after clinical disease (Jama 1958;200:365); occasionally parenteral; higher incidence in parents of day care center children, children are often asx (Nejm 1980;302:1222)

In travelers to developing countries, 3/1000/mo incidence for first-class hotel users, 20/1000/mo for community living guests; thus is most frequent preventable infection in travelers (Jama 1994;272:885)

Only in humans; because it is an enterovirus, incidence up in late summer and early winter; 45% of adults have had it (Nejm 1976;95:755); increased incidence in gay males (Nejm 1980;302:438)

Risk for travelers: From 3–20/1000 per month among nonimmune travelers in developing countries

Incubation period: 15–40 d

Sx: In children, only 5–15% get sx

Malaise (48% in children/63% in adults), anorexia (41%/42%), abdominal pain (48%/37%), fever and/or chills (41%/32%), jaundice (65%/88%), diarrhea (58%/18%), dark urine (58%/68%), light stools (58%/58%), nausea and vomiting (65%/26%)

Si: Jaundice, though anicteric form also common and more benign

Crs: Often benign, 15% morbidity but rare (0.3%) mortality (Ann IM 1998;128:111); sx peak 2 wk after onset and take about 4 wk to clear; relapse in 6% at 1–3 mo (Ann IM 1987;106:221)

Cmplc: Fulminant hepatitis, relapsing hepatitis (no chronic active hepatitis); r/o Q fever, EBV, CMV, toxoplasmosis, Fitzhugh–Curtis syndrome, psittacosis, and other viral hepatitis (20.7, 20.9, 20.10), esp hepatitis E, which is spread via water sources esp in equatorial areas (Virol 1993;4:273) and in pregnant women

Lab:

Chem: typical hepatitis enzyme picture w ALT (SGPT) > AST (SGOT) > LDH > alkaline phos levels

Serol: hepatitis A IgM antibody present when first sx present (Ann IM 1982;96:193); later IgM goes negative and IgG appears and stays

Rx: (Ann IM 1985;103:391)

Prevent: Avoid fecal contamination; vaccine, inactivated (Havrix or Vaqta) (Nejm 1997;336:197, Med Let 1995;37:51; Jama 1995;273:906; 1994;272:885; Nejm 1992;327:453) 2-shot (1 cc w 1440 ELU im) series for adults 6–12 (see 3.9) mo apart, 3-shot (0.55 cc, 720 ELU im) series for children at 0, 1 mo, and 6–12 mo; 100% effective, no need to screen titers if born after 1945, may be useful postexposure (80% efficacy) (Lancet 1999;353:1136) but not clearly better than IgG (ACP J Club 1999;131:45), often will need to prophylax w IgG 0.02 cc/kg up to 2 cc im if exposed of disease, bed rest probably no benefit (Nejm 1969;281:193)

20.8 HEPATITIS B

Nejm 1997;337:1733, Ann IM 1980;93:165

Cause: Hepatitis B virus; genetic susceptibility at least for carrier states? (Nejm 1973;289:1162)

Epidem: Worldwide, but highly endemic in parts of SE Asia, China, Africa, the Pacific (Fig. 3.4); primarily spread venereally or via blood and blood products in U.S. (transfusion risk = 1/63,000, Nejm 1996;334:1685), fresh, dry, or frozen (Nejm 1978;298:637) (eg, communal autolet in hospitals; Nejm 1992;326:721);

transmitted by mucous membranes but not by urine and feces (Nejm 1969;281:1375); and via eczematous skin (Ann IM 1976;85:573)

Risk for travelers: Low, except w sexual contact, unsterile needles, etc.; risk is an important consideration in long-term visitors, expatriates, etc.

Incubation period: 60–120 d

Pathophys: Sometimes viral DNA incorporated into liver genome, then less hepatitis, but still can produce hep BsAg, associated with carcinoma more often? (Nejm 1986;315:1187)

Sx: Arthralgias/arthritis (Ann IM 1971;74:207; 1971;75:29; Nejm 1978;298:185), cryoglobulins (Ann IM 1977;87:287), urticaria and other rashes (Ann IM 1978;89:34)

Si: Many cases anicteric

Crs: Acute hepatitis, leads to:
- Benign course, recover or have relapsing, or mild portal hepatitis; or
- Acute liver necrosis, all of whom die w/o transplant; or
- Submassive hepatic necrosis (bridging), of whom 60% die or go on to postnecrotic cirrhosis
- The balance recover completely; or
- Chronic active hepatitis, usually with a progressive downhill course over 5–10 yr; or
- Asx carrier state in ~90% newborns, 20% school age children, <1% young healthy adults (WWII vaccine epidemic, Nejm 1987;316:965)

Cmplc: Hepatoma; chronic active hepatitis (10%); delta (d) agent infection (hepatitis D), an RNA viral parasite of hep B virus, only can replicate if hep B around, leads to acute hepatitis itself or severe chronic active hepatitis (Nejm 1987;317:1256), hep B carriers get it from subsequent transfusions (Nejm 1985;312:1488, 1515); fasting hypoglycemia (Nejm 1972;286:1436); serum sickness (20%), polyarteritis, nephritis (Bull Rheum Dis 1983;33:16), esp membranous GN (Nejm 1991;324:1457)

Lab:

Chem: typical hepatitis enzyme picture w ALT (SGPT) > AST (SGOT) > LDH > alkaline phos levels; get CPK to r/o myopathy if LDH > AST (SGOT) > ALT (SGPT)

Path: liver bx, consider if not improving in 2–3 wk

Serol: core IgM antibody always up by time of first sx (Nejm 1978;298:1379); HBsAg (Ann IM 1982;96:193) elevated; e-antigen elevation correlates with infectivity; anti-HBsAg appears shortly after sx develop, but there may be a window of infectivity when HBsAg and antibody is negative but core (c) antibody is positive which, if IgM, can be distinguished from remote infection w attenuation of all but IgG core antibody

Rx: (Ann IM 1985;103:391)

Prevent:

- Body fluid precautions including wearing gloves (Ann IM 1981;95:133)
- Monitor hep B pos health workers but let work unless surgeons doing high exposure surgery, then should not work if hep B e Ag positive or documented transmissions (Nejm 1997;336:178)
- Screen all pregnant women for HBsAg (Ann IM 1987;107:412) so can prophylax and immunize their infants
- Hep B immune globulin (HBIG) prophylaxis 0.05 cc/kg × 2, 30 d apart within 24–72 h of exposure (Nejm 1980;303:833; Med Let 1978;20:9); for newborns of HBsAg pos mothers 0.5 cc within 12 h of birth (Nejm 1985;313:1398) along w vaccine
- Immunization w recombinant vaccine (Nejm 1997;336:196; Med Let 1985;27:118; Ann IM 1982;97:379, 362); cmplc: rare post-vaccine alopecia (Jama 1997;278:1176), possibly incr in later autoimmune disease
- Adults/children w 20 mgm q 1 mo × 2 then 3rd dose in 6–12 mo, or q 1 yr × 3 doses also work (Rx Let 1999;6:38); $100; neither vaccine nor HBIG necessary if anti-HBc present, but are needed if only anti-HBsAg (Ann IM 1985;103:21, 201)
- Newborns, all w 10 mgm at birth, 1 and 6 mo (Jama 1995;274:1201) esp to SE Asian children to prevent 7% incidence of child-to-child transmisssion (Jama 1996;276:906; Nejm 1989;321:1301); for newborns of HBsAg pos mothers (Med Let 1992;34:69), vaccinate and give HBIG as above
- Vaccination has halved Taiwan rate of childhood hepatoma (Nejm 1997;336:1855) of disease, to prevent cirrhosis progression and/or hepatoma: interferon-$\alpha 2\alpha$ or 2β × 4–6 mo may permanently help 30–40% if given early on, certainly for chronic d-agent infection (Nejm 1994;330:88), and for chronic hep B (Nejm 1994;330:137), esp if e-antigen pos (Nejm 1996;334:1422; Ann IM 1995;122:664)
- Lamivudine (3TC) 100$^+$ mg po qd × 1 yr (Nejm 1999;341:1256; 1998;339:61, 114), but resistance develops so multidrug regimens being developed (Ann IM 2000;132:723)
- No steroids (Nejm 1976;294:722)

20.9 HEPATITIS C

Jama 1997;277:1268; Ann IM 2000;132:296; Nejm 1992;327:1899;
    1989;321:1494, 1501

Cause: Hepatitis C RNA virus, several genotypes, 1a and 1b most
    common in U.S.; causes 82% of nonA nonB hepatitis; but not
    present in fulminant nonA nonB hepatitis (Ann IM 1991;115:111)
    except for one report (Nejm 1996;335:635)

Epidem: Worldwide; 1.4% prevalence of antibodies in the U.S., 4
    million infected (Nejm 1999;341:556), but up to 5%+ in Africa
    and Middle East; over 50% of cases due to iv drug use; 50–80%
    of iv drug users contract within first yr of use. 97% of post-
    transfusion hepatitis in U.S. (Nejm 1991;325:1325); transfusions,
    incidence = 1/100,000 transfusions using screened blood
    (Nejm 1996;334:1685), 18/10,000 using unscreened blood
    (Nejm 1992;327:369); Post-organ transplant (eg, renal; Nejm
    1992;326:454); sexual transmission rates are low but real
    (eg, 2–3% annual incidence in wives of infected hemophiliacs;
    Ann IM 1994;120:748; 1991;115:764)

Neonatal transmission rate low, 2.5% (Ann IM 1992;117:881,
    887) to 5% (Nejm 1994;330:744) as is intrafamilial rate (Jama
    1995;274:1459); chronic carrier state develops in 85%+ after
    acute infection and lasts years even with normal LFTs (Nejm
    1992;327:1899); 90% with hep C antibody have infectious blood
    (Nejm 1990;323:1107)

Pathophys: No protective antibody response develops

Incubation period: 2–20 wk, 6–7 wk average

Sx: Often asymptomatic until late disease

Si: Often none unless cirrhosis, etc.

Crs: 17+ yr after infection, 80%+ had fatigue, all had at least mild
    inflammation on bx, 55% had pos enzymes, but only 2% had
    cirrhosis (Jama 2000;284:450; Nejm 1999;340:1228); vs 11%
    of HCV pos army recruits eventually got liver disease over 45 yr
    (Ann IM 2000;132:105)

Acute hepatitis, leads to:

- Chronic active hepatitis in most (see below), or
- Benign course, recover or have relapsing, or mild/portal hepatitis; or
- Acute liver necrosis, all of whom die w/o transplant; or

- Submassive hepatic necrosis (bridging), of whom 60% die or go on to postnecrotic cirrhosis
- The balance recover completely

Cmplc: Mixed cryoglobulinemia

CHRONIC ACTIVE HEPATITIS in 80% over 10⁺ yr, 20–35% of whom go on to cirrhosis over 20 yr; hepatocellular carcinoma over 30 yr, mostly via cirrhosis induction and independent of hep B (Ann IM 1992;116:97); get CPK, esp if LDH > AST (SGOT) > ALT (SGPT) to r/o myopathy

Liver bix (do if sx beyond 6–12 mo or worsening) shows fibrosis with bridging between hepatic lobules but pathologic picture waxes and wanes; r/o other causes of chronically elevated LFTs: hemochromatosis, Wilson's disease, α_1-antitrypsin deficiency (Nejm 1981;304:558), Aldomet-induced hepatitis, oxyphenisatin laxative induction (Nejm 1971;285:813), NSAIDs (Med Let 1983;25:15), primary biliary cirrhosis, alcohol and other toxins, diabetes, myxedema, myopathies; r/o other nonA nonB hepatitis, such as HEPATITIS E virus infection, an enterovirus that causes only acute mild hepatitis similar to hep A (Nejm 1997;336:795); and HEPATITIS G, rare, perhaps benign, blood borne (Nejm 1997;336:741, 747, 795; Ann IM 1997;126:874)

Lab:

Chem: Elevated LFTs, esp SGPT (ALT), but not 100% sens (Ann IM 1995;123:330)

Serol: Anti-hep C virus IgG antibody levels (ELISA with RIBA f/u) first detectable 10–50 wk after transfusion and 4–50 wk after LFT elevations appear; hep C viral RNA correlates with infectivity and persistence as chronic active hepatitis (Nejm 1991;325:98), tested for by PCR method or more inconsistent branched-chain DNA PCR assay (Ann IM 1995;123:321)

Rx: (Mmwr 1998;47:RR-19)

Prevent: Avoid high-risk behaviors (iv drugs, sexual promiscuity), body fluid precautions, and by screening and rejecting donor blood with hep B core antibody and/or elevated aminotransferases (AST [SGOT]); will eliminate 3% of all donor blood and prevent 20–30% of nonA nonB posttransfusion hepatitis (Nejm 1987; 317:137). Screening donors for anti-HCV levels will prevent 60% (Nejm 1990;323:1107) to 85% of cases; a small % of donors will be infectious but won't yet be antibody positive

Prophylaxis with immune globulin is ineffective in disease (elevated ALT, viremia and cirrhosis on bx); decr incidence of hepatoma (Ann IM 1998;129:94); much more effective in the 25% w a susceptibility gene (Nejm 1996;334:77); NIH and CDC suggest checking ALT and RNA levels after 6 mo rx and stopping if not markedly improved (Ann IM 1997;127:855, 866, 918; Hepatol 1996;24:778); may decr cancer incidence 50%[+] (Ann IM 1999;131:174); can reverse cirrhotic fibrosis (Ann IM 2000;132:517) w:

- Interferon-α2β 3 million U sc tiw × 24–52 wk, and other α interferons (Jama 1998;280:2088); helps half improve LFTs, but 50%[+] relapse after rx, then retreat combined w
- Ribavirin (Med Lct 1999;41:53; Am J Med 1999;107:112; Lancet 1998;352:1426) × 6–12 mos, more side effects and $8000/6 mo, but helps another 50% cost effectively (Am J Med 2000;108:366); other options: liver transplant; lamivudine (3TC) possibly at 100[+] mg pq qd (Nejm 1995;333:1657); hep A vaccination if not immune already, to prevent frequently fatal hep A infection of chronic hep C hepatitis (Nejm 1998;338:286)

20.10 HEPATITIS E

Epidemiologic Rev 1999;21:162

Cause: RNA virus, closely related to calicivirus

Epidem: Worldwide; predom Asia, no Africa, Mexico; estimated 2 million cases/yr in India; rare in developed countries; fecal–oral transmission; waterborne outbreaks, partic after flooding (Lancet 2000;354:1050); mortality rate 0.5–4%, incr to 20% in pregnant women

Risk for travelers: May be significant in some areas, but seroconversion appears rare in travelers (Am J Trop Med Hyg 1995;53:233); most cases in Israeli travelers acquired in Indian subcontinent (CID; 1999;29:1312); asymptomatic infx may occur in 1% of travel clinic pts spending time in tropics (Am J Trop Med Hyg 1999;61:822)

Pathogen: Viremia × 14 d, w viral shedding to 6 wk

Incubation period: 16–60 d (average 40 d)

Sx: Fever, jaundice, dark urine, light stools, abd pain

Si: Fever, jaundice, hepatomegaly

Crs: Usually self-limited (many infx may be w/o sx); incr mortality w prgnancy as noted above

Lab: Incr LFTs (usually cholestatic) for 4–5 wks, may persist 90 d

    Serol: hep E ELISA (may not be routinely available); contact Hepatitis Branch of CDC (404-639-3048); antibodies may not be detectable for several wks to mos after infx

Rx: Supportive

Prevent: Food–water precautions; avoid travel to high-risk areas in pregnancy; vaccine trial is underway

20.11 HIV/ACQUIRED IMMUNE DEFICIENCY SYNDROME (AIDS)

Cause: Human immunodeficiency virus (HIV) type 1 (Nejm 1991;324:308); HIV 2 rarely in U.S. but commonly in W Africa (Ann IM 1993;118:211); both retroviruses

Epidem: Worldwide; highest prevalence in SubSaharan Africa—up to 1/3 adults (15–49) infected; up to 80% of boys age 15 now predicted to die of AIDS in some African countries; rapid incr in Asia, Eastern Europe

Spread via sex (3% infection rate w HIV pos semen; Jama 1995;273:854); dirty/shared needles; blood products (eg, screened blood transfusion 1996 risk = 1/500,000; Nejm 1996;334:1685), factor VIII concentrates (Nejm 1993;329:1835; 1984;310:69), and probably breast milk (Nejm 1991;325:593); percutaneous inoculation in health care workers, 0.3%/incident, incr w incr volume and probably HIV titer (Nejm 1997;337:1485)

Transmission enhanced by the presence of chancroid or other genital ulcers (Ann IM 1993;119:1150), may account for higher rates of heterosexual spread in Africa, Haiti, etc., as may difference in subtypes (in U.S./Europe, mostly subtype B; others in Africa, Asia)

HIV 1 subtypes differ geographically; some (ie, subtype E) may be assoc w higher risk heterosex transmission; incidence of AIDS in late 1990s decr in U.S. as are AIDS deaths, probably from preventive maneuvers, drug rx of HIV infection, and prophylaxis and rx of opportunistic infections (Mmwr 1997;46:861)

Risk for travelers: Primarily from unprotected sex contact or parenteral drug use; possible w use of unsterilized needle for injections or blood transfusion, though blood supply protected in most areas; 1 case of apparent transmission after traumatic blood contact; note that epidem studies reveal higher risk sex behavior among some groups (ic, U.S. college students, Peace Corps, others) during travel (see AIDS 1995;9:795; 1994;8:247)

Pathophys: AIDS defined by HIV infection and T4 count <200; increased suppressor T8 and decreased helper T4 cells (CD4) (Nejm 1985;313:79); deficient production of interferon-γ (Nejm 1985;313:1504); billions of virions produced daily from infection w high viral RNA mutation rate, which allows rapid selection of resistant organisms in face of rx (Ann IM 1996;124:984)

Sx: Primary HIV infection (Nejm 1998;339:33; Ann IM 1996;125:259) consists of a mono-like syndrome 5–30 d after exposure lasting ~2 wk, rarely seek care; w fever (95%), sore throat (70%), weight loss (70%), myalgias (60%), headache (60%), cervical adenopathy (50%), maculopapular or other rash involving trunk (40–80%)

AIDS: diarrhea (60%; Nejm 1993;329:14), malaise, weight loss, fever, adenopathy, dyspnea (pneumocystis pneumonia)

Si:

Early: lymphadenopathy; oral monilia/thrush (exudative, chelosis or erythematous diffuse rash types) precedes overt disease often (Nejm 1984;311:354); dermatoses including warts and shingles; chronic fatigue syndrome

Later: wasting syndromes, chronic diarrhea, dementias/seizures, FUO, thrombocytopenia, cervical dysplasia, Kaposi's sarcoma, hairy leukoplakia corrugations on sides of tongue due to reactivation of EBV (Nejm 1985;313:1564)

Crs: Variable RNA viral loads in first 4 mo but worse crs predicted by levels at 5–12 mo from infection and by severity of primary infection sx (Ann IM 1998;128:613)

Rx: *HIV infection:* Evolution to AIDS 10 yr post seroconversion varies from 0–72% inversely w RNA copies (viral load) at 12–18 mo after seroconversion (Jama 1996;276:105)

AIDS: 1997 mortality figures markedly improving w aggressive multidrug rx based on viral loads (Jama 1998;279:450) (eg, from 29 to 9/100 person years in pts w CD4 counts <100 (Nejm 1998;338:853); older data were 50% 1-yr, 15% 5-yr survival (Nejm 1987;317:1297), 5% 10+ yr survival because of some viral attenuated pathogenicity (Nejm 1995;332:201, 217); in pts w AIDS on AZT, 50% 1-yr survival after CD4 count <50/mm³. Prognosis (survival) worse w increasing age of pt, but not associated w gender, iv drug use, race, or socioeconomic status (Nejm 1995;333:751); note that progression of HIV 2 is slower than HIV 1

Cmplc:

- Infections with common bacterial pathogens (Nejm 1995;333:845) as well as opportunistic organisms esp when CD4 <50 (Ann IM 1996;124:333) including: *Pneumocystis* (in 1980s was presenting sx in 75%, now much rarer w prophylaxis; Nejm 1993;329:1822), atypical mycobacteria (Ann IM 1986;105:184), especially *M. avium/intracellulare*, rarely *M. haemophilum* (Ann IM 1994;120:118) (see 16.2); herpes infections including tongue fissures (Nejm 1993;329:1859); CMV; candida; aspergillosis; cryptococcus (17.3), esp meningitis; toxoplasma encephalitis, cryptosporidiosis (18.11), *Isospora belli* (18.2), listeria (Nejm 1985;312:404), cat scratch *Bartonella (Rochalimaea) henselae* or *quintana* causing bacillary angiomatosis (r/o Kaposi's by bx) and peliosis hepatitis (16.10, 16.48)
- Syphilis w rapid (<4 yr) appearance of neurosyphilis manifest by strokes, meningitis, and cranial nerve palsies and which is only transiently suppressed by penicillin regimens (Nejm 1994;331:1469, 1488, 1516); see 16.44
- Geographic exposure assoc w partic opportunistic infections; *Penicillium* infx in SE Asia (17.7); Chagas (18.9), paracoccidioidomycosis in Latin America (17.6); kala-azar in Mediterranean areas (18.24); dissem cocci in sw U.S. (17.2), dissem histo in mid-U.S. (17.4); isosporiasis in Carribean (18.2)

NOTE: High prevalence of coinfection w tbc in some groups, esp SubSaharan Africa, Haiti

- Tumors including:

KAPOSI'S SARCOMA

Cause: human herpes 8 virus (HHV-8) coinfection (Nejm 1998;338:948; 1997;336:163; 1996;334:1168, 1292; Jama 1997;277:478)

Epidem: HHV-8 is venereally spread, at least among gay males

Sx + Si: Violaceous skin eruptions, ulcers on legs, r/o angiomatosis (see above)

Cmplc:
- R/o bacillary angiomatosis by bx
- Hematologic including ITP (Nejm 1985;313:1375) and aplastic anemias from parvovirus infections (Ann IM 1990;113:926); and from diminished half-life and megakaryocyte infection (Nejm 1992;327:1779)
- Myocardiopathy (Nejm 1992;327:1260)
- Neurologic (Ann IM 1994;121:769) including early subtle CNS degeneration (Nejm 1990;323:864) leading to dementia (Nejm 1995;332:934; Ann IM 1987;107:383); progressive multifocal leukoencephalopathy (Ann IM 1987;107:78) associated w papovavirus, seen in transplant pts as well, cytarabine rx no help (Nejm 1998;338:1345); cord lesions; aseptic meningitis; peripheral neuropathy (Nejm 1985;313:1538); cerebral toxoplasmosis; cerebral lymphomas; nephropathy (Nejm 1989;321:625)
- Rheumatologic including Reiter's without conjunctivitis; and psoriasis with arthritis (Bull Rheum Dis 990;39:5)
- Suicide (Jama 1996;276:1743)
- r/o HTLV I and II infections, former associated w paraparesis, latter w no disease (Ann IM 1993;118:448); rare idiopathic CD4 cell lymphopenia syndrome (Nejm 1993;328:429)

Lab:

Immunol: (Med Let 1997;39:81)
- Viral load, most important test, positive at >50,000/cc in acute primary disease (Nejm 1998;339:33); RNA by PCR, peripheral mononuclear cell viral m-RNA levels predict prognosis (Ann IM 1995;123:641) and treatment success (Nejm 1996;335:1091, 1996;334:426; Ann IM 1996;124:984); indicates rapidity of disease progression (Jama 1997;278:983); <10,000/cc good, 10,000–100,000/cc moderately ok, >100,000/cc bad
- NOTE that pts w non-subtype B HIV infx (ie, most Africans, Asians) may have unobtainable viral load by current PCR; bDNA test of viral load may give more accurate result; subgroup O infx (W Africa) may not be detected by either
- T4 (CD4) <200/cc defines AIDS now (Mmwr 1992;41(RR-17):1) and predicts opportunistic pneumonias (Ann IM 1989;111:223); 200–500 = intermediate risk (Nejm 1989;321:1141); a form of mile marker in disease progression (Jama 1997;278:983)
- ELISA, only 1.5% false positive in low-risk military population (Nejm 1988;319:961); 5% false pos in blood donors when Western

blot lacks p31 band (Jama 1998;280:1080); combined two-step
ELISA/WB falsely pos in <1/100,000 (Am J Med 2000;109:575);
if indeterminant, repeat in 1 mo and should become pos if
really HIV 1; if persistently equivocal, get PCR and viral culture;
consider HIV 2, tests negative for 4+ mo incubation period (Nejm
1989;321:941); NOTE that not all ELISA tests screen for HIV 2,
and Western blot often indeterminate/neg; subgroup O of HIV 1
(W Africa) also not detected by some screens (Am J Med
2000;109:575)
- Ora-Sure HIV-1 test from 2 min swab btwn cheek and gum, as
specific as serum by ELISA/Western Blot (Jama 1997;277:254)

Rx: (Nejm 1995;333:450; 1993;328:1686)

Preventive maneuvers: Universal precautions (guidelines; Ann
IM 1986;105:730); risk is very low, even with needle sticks
(Nejm 1985;312:1); screen blood donors with ELISA test (Nejm
1989;321:917, 941, 947, 966); consistent condom use prevents
disease; 0/124 conversions in HIV neg partners over 2 yr,
otherwise 5/100 pt/yr convert (Nejm 1994;331:341)

In infants (Nejm 1995;333:298) avoid peripartum scalp
electrodes, breast feeding, rupture of membranes >4 hr (Nejm
1996;334:1617), and episiotomies. Pre- and peripartum AZT
no matter what the maternal viral load or CD4 count (Nejm
1996;335:1621) reduces maternal–fetal transmission from 25%
to 8% (Nejm 1994;331:1173); rx of prepartum mother viral load
to <20,000, infant infection rate = 0 (Jama 1996;275:599)

Prophylaxis immediately postexposure × 1 mo w AZT (Nejm
1997;337:1485) + lamivudine (3TC) (Ann IM 1998;128:306;
Jama 1996;276:146) or w 3-drug regimens as per CDC

Prevention of AIDS-associated infections (Jama 1998;279:130;
and USPHS comprehensive and tabular)

See also recent guidelines (Jama 2000;283:381)

20.12 HTLV 1 (TROPICAL SPASTIC PARAPARESIS)

Guerrant Trop Inf Dis, 1999, ch 121:1301

Cause: Retroviruses of the HTLV-BLV group; HTLV 1 has 65% genetic homology w HIV 1; may cause adult T-cell leukemia (ATL) or myelopathy (TSP)

Epidem: HTLV 1 endemic in Carribean, Japan (prevalence reaches 35% on Okinawa), equatorial Africa, Papua New Guinea, E Asia; Also in ivDUs in Europe, U.S.; transmission is person–person by sexual contact, blood transfusion, needles, etc. as w HIV

Risk for travelers: Low, but focally high prevalence in some populations suggests risk for travelers who engage in unprotected sexual contact or ivDU

Incubation period: Mo to yr for development of myelopathy or ATL; post-transfusion of HTLV 1 infected blood, shortest time to myelopathy was 18 wk (Nejm 1990; 322:383); average of 20–30 yrs from infx to ATL

Sx: Lymphoma is indolent w fever, weight loss, rash, abd pain; myelopathy, slowly progressive bilat paralysis of LEs

Si: Hepatomegaly, lymphadenopathy, arthritis, skin lesions

Crs: Indolent smoldering leukemia to rapid disease w death in 8 mo

Lab: Abnormal lymphocytes on peripheral smear; eosinophilia; hypercalcemia; dx w viral isolation or antibody detection

Rx: Unknown

Prevent: Avoid sexual contact w infected persons; screen blood

20.13 LASSA FEVER

Nejm 1990;323:1120; 1986;314:20

Cause: Lassa fever virus, an arenavirus

Epidem: W Africa, villages; endemic in Sierra Leone (300,000 cases/yr in Africa); accounts for 30% of hospital deaths in E Sierra Leone (Wilson, 1991); most common during dry season, when rat reservoir host (*Mastomys natalensis*) enters villages; transmission by contact w rodent fomites, feces, urine; spread also by contact w infected fluids of pts; person–person/nosocomial spread rare, as is aerosol (BMJ 1995;311:857)

Risk for travelers: Rare, though living in rural village houses in Sierra Leone would be a risk; <1% of expatriate missionaries in W Africa seropositive (Wilson, 1991)

Pathophys: Incr capillary fragility leads to bleeding

Incubation period: 7–18 d

Sx: Fever, sore throat, back pain, cough, ha, abd pain

Si: Pharyngitis, often exudative; conjunctivitis; rare rash

Crs: 1–4 wks, 15–20% mortality in hosp pts; 53% mort w/o rx, 5% w rx

Cmplc: GI hemorrhage, hypovolemic shock; ARDS; encephalopathy; pericarditis; CHF; sensorineural deafness

Dx: Combination of fever, pharyngitis, retrosternal pain, proteinuria in endemic area has predictive value positive of 80% (Wilson, 1991)

Lab:

Chem: aspartate aminotransferease (AST) = 150 IU/mL; other LFTs also incr; proteinuria present

Serol: Combined ELISA for IgM antibody/antigen has sens 90% (J Clin Microbiol 1984;20:239)

Rx: Call CDC; strict isolation in hospitals (Mmwr 1988;314:20); ribavirin iv/po (30 mg/kg initially, then 15 mg/kg q 6 hr × 4 d, then 7.5 mg/kg q 8 hr × 6 d); (see Nejm 1986;314:20)

Prevent: Avoid direct rodent contact or contract w infected areas; health care workers should use strict precautions (incl aerosol)

20.14 POLIOMYELITIS

Cause: Polio virus, an enterovirus

Epidem: Residual foci in Asia/Africa; eradicated from W hemisphere in 1997 (but outbreak in Dominican Republic in 2000 w reversion of vaccine-related strain to wild type); fecal–oral spread; peak incidence in summer and fall; paradoxically occurs in countries with good sewage systems; correlates inversely with infant mortality, when <70/1000, many persons not infected in infancy when protected with maternal antibody and hence are susceptible when older, when the disease is much more damaging; increased clinical incidence in pregnant or ovulating females; after T + A bulbar polio is increased, even if T + A was years ago (only 0.1–1% cases show clinical si (ie, most are subclinical; most cases now acquired outside of U.S. in persons immunized as children or as vaccine-associated; see below)

Risk for travelers: Generally very low, and becoming lower w continued global efforts at eradication; vaccinated travelers w/o booster in adulthood at risk of polio due to declining antibodies as are unvaccinated individuals

Pathophys: Hits anterior horn cells and sympathetic ganglia; starts in GI reticuloendothelial system; inhibits RNA polymerase

Incubation period: 6–18 d

Sx: Fever, malaise, drowsy, headache, nausea, diarrhea or constipation, sore throat; may have stiff neck, low-back pain

Si: An aseptic meningitis; meningismus for 2–10 d; flaccid paralysis, maximum in a few days, maximum recovery in 6 mo; spinal type may be in muscles of lumbar, dorsal, or cervical areas; bulbar type in upper (CN III–VIII), lower (CN IX–XII), or medullary (immediate threat to life)

Crs: 6–18 d incubation period; death in 15% if patient >15 yr old; in 2.5% if patient <15 yr

Cmplc: Encephalitis; viral pneumonia; late post-polio muscular atrophy due to reactivated CNS infection (Nejm 1991;325:749) w partial motor neuron dysfunction and dropout but not total dropout (Nejm 1987;317:7; 1986;314:959) including dysphagia from bulbar involvement (Nejm 1991;324:1162) r/o other causes of "viral" meningitis: Coxsackie, echo, viral hepatitis, leptospirosis, et al.

Lab:

CSF: Aseptic meningitis picture

Serol: Comp-fix, and neutralizing antibody titers

Prevent: (Ann IM 1982;96:630)

Gamma globulin for passive, short-lived protection

Vaccine: eIPV; killed virus, lasts 6+ yr; 70% effective; in adults (eg, travelers), boost with inactivated enhanced polio vaccine (eIPV); avoids rare risk (1/several million) of vaccine-acquired polio, and risk to immunosuppressed household contacts

Sabin (Nejm 1977;297:249), live attenuated, 90% effective, spreads to other intimate contacts, elicits GI RES secretory IgA immunity as well as systemic unlike Salk (Nejm 1968;279:893); give in winter to avoid interferon of other enteroviruses? can itself induce

clinical polio in 1/2,000,000 adults (Jama 1967;201:771)
(eg, adult family members of children being immunized, in
immunocompromised patients, or in pts given im injections of
anything w/i 30 d of oral polio vaccine; Nejm 1995;332:500);
possibly a mixture of 2 doses of Salk then 2 doses of Sabin
vaccine (Jama 1996;276:967)

20.15 RABIES

Ann IM 1998;128:922; Nejm 1993;329:1632; CID 2000;30:4
Cause: Rabies virus, one of 7 serotypes of *Lyssavirus*
Epidem: Worldwide; (see section 3, Table 3.9). 50,000 or more deaths
per yr; highest risk India (30,000 cases/yr); SE Asia; Africa
From saliva of infected animal, inhaling infected guano in bat caves,
or corneal transplants (Nejm 1979;300:603); bats may be reservoir
since not killed by it; cats are now most commonly affected
domestic animal in U.S.; dogs in developing countries; most
common wild animals affected: bats, foxes, skunks, raccoons; and
prey species like rabbits, woodchucks, and goats; cyclic prevalence
q 100 yr, peaked in 1965; 20 cases in U.S. 1960–1980 (Ann IM
1984;100:728); incr again in U.S. so that 22 cases 1990–1996
Risk for travelers: High rates of dog rabies in some urban areas;
problem in unvaccinated (ie, w/o preexposure vaccine) travelers to
remote areas may be access to effective vaccine, esp RIG; only 3%
of courses of postexposure prophylaxis in Thailand received RIG
(CID 1998;27:751); 1–2%/yr of long-term travelers may suffer
animal bite but rabies in U.S. travelers have been rare; risk from
single rabid bite 30–50% (Wilson, 1991)
Pathophys: Initially cell free in wound; then spreads along nerves to
CNS (viral spread at 1–40 cm/d); leads to eventual inhibition of
neurotransmitters (Negri bodies on path), hypothalamic damage
Incubation period: 20–60 d; possible range of 6 d to >6 mo
Sx: H/o animal bite, except in bat rabies, where often no h/o bite
or even bat contact (Mmwr 1995;44:625); pain/paresthesias at
exposure site in 50%; in 2–10 d, difficulty swallowing in 65%;
fever; nausea and vomiting; Guillain-Barré-like syndrome;
in hyperactive form, agitation, confusion, hydrophobia,

hypersalivation, seizures, priapism; in paralytic form, peripheral
nerve dysfunction (ascending paralysis), confusion, fever

Si: Encephalitis with tonic contractions of muscles, esp throat on
minimal stimulation (hence hydrophobia); flaccid paralysis

Crs: 15–60 d incubation (depends on nerve length), rarely up to 6 yr
later (Nejm 1991;324:205); Fatal unless rx before sx, usually,
although some severe cases now recovering with supportive care
(ie, respirator, etc; Ann IM 1976;85:44); 2/38 survived 1960–1980

Cmplc: May be misdiagnosed as Guillain-Barré syndrome (in GBS, have
sensory sx, less fever, normal mentation)

Lab: Dx w RT PCR of saliva (100% sens), nuchal skin bx for rabies;
Ag (60–70% sens); brain bx (IFA, ELISA)

CSF: Elevated protein after 1 wk; cells are a mix of lymphs and
polys, 6–300/mm^3

Path: Negri bodies in brain at post

Serol: Half positive after 1 wk of sx, 2/3 after 1–1/2 wk, all positive
by 2 wk of sx

Rx: Supportive.

Prevent: Vaccinate (Med Let 1998;40:64) w human diploid cell vaccine
(HDCV) (Imovax); rabies vaccine absorbed, or purified chick
embryo cell (PCEC) (RabAvert); all ~$700/5 shot series;
chloroquine malaria prophylaxis may prevent adequate
immunization (Nejm 1986;314:280)

- Primary series postexposure = HDCV im on day 1, 3, 7, 14, 28
  (PLUS HRIG, or in foreign areas, if HRIG not available, use equine
  RIG—1% risk serum sickness)
- Preexposure = day 1, 7, and 28 im, or 1/10 im dose id day 1, 7, 21,
  or 28; do not use id route w chloroquine or mefloquine prophylaxis
  as concurrent use may decr immune response to vaccine (use im
  route in this event)
- Booster-post repeat exposure after previous primary series w shots
  day 0 and 3 q 2 yr to veterinarians and other high-risk people, or
  follow titer q yr and boost if <0.5 IU
- For acute single exposure: wash wound; vaccinate as above + HRIG
  (immune globulin) 20 IU/kg, 1/2 in wound, 1/2 im in deltoid in
  adult, thigh in child, not gluteal area (Nejm 1987;316:1256,
  1270); use liberally even if no bite in bat exposures
  (Mmwr 1999;48(RR1):1)

20.16 YELLOW FEVER

Jama 1996;276:1157; Guerrant Trop Inf Dis 1999; ch 116:1253

Cause: Yellow fever virus, an arbovirus of the flavivirus group

Epidem: Tropical Africa and South America (10 N–25 S); vector is the mosquito, *Aedes aegypti* in urban settings; in rainforest, canopy dwelling mosquitos (*Haemagogus* sp.) maintain cycle in primates; in Africa, *Aedes africanus* maintains at jungle-savannah interface w occasional epidemic spread into savannah areas; risk incr w rainy season or following it; ecological factors favor reemergence in some urban areas; recent outbreak in Bolivian city of Santa Cruz (Lancet 1999;353:1558); humans are only reservoirs in urban cycle, monkeys in jungle cycle; increasing problem in Africa and So America; est 1 million people infx in Nigeria in past decade; could reappear in so U.S. where *A. aegypti* is endemic

Risk for travelers: Rare, but most travelers to endemic areas receive vaccine, which is highly effective; several recent deaths in unvaccinated travelers reported (Mmwr 2000;49:303) underscore importance of vaccination for travelers to risk areas

Pathophys: Viremia and coagulative necrosis of liver w Councilman's bodies

Incubation period: 3–14 d

Sx: Malaise, nonspecific febrile illness w myalgias, ha, back pain followed (in severe cases) in 3–4 d by jaundice, renal failure, DIC; sometimes a biphasic illness

Si: Icterus; tender liver; fever >105°F (40.5°C); facial/conjunctival congestion; red furred tongue; relative bradycardia; r/o viral hepatitis, salmonella, malaria, leptospirosis, gram-negative shock, psittacosis, rickettsial, Q fever, other viral hemorrhagic fever

Crs: 10–15% mortality, 50% mortality if reach toxic icteric phase

Cmplc: Hepatic or renal failure, myocarditis; r/o dengue (Jama 1997;277:1546, Nejm 1989;321:957), mosquito-transmitted febrile illness often with exanthematous rash, usually benign course, possibly helped by vaccination vs Japanese encephalitis (Nejm 1988;319:808)

Lab:

    Chem: Elevated LFTs; leukopenia; eventual DIC

    Path: Liver bx shows viral hepatitis picture but more irregular necrosis and Councilman's bodies, which are questionably distinguishable from Mallory's bodies?

    Serol: IgM antibodies (ELISA, antigen capture); culture (in mouse)

Rx: Supportive

Prevent: In epidemics, by spraying to kill mosquitos if >5–10% homes have Aedes; travelers should use DEET-containing repellants; note that these mosquitos are day biting

    Vaccine, live virus; effective in 1 wk; use in endemic areas (eg, So America and Africa); 1/2 cc sc; lasts 10⁺ yr; egg base (Ann IM 1969;71:365); available at special distribution centers in U.S. (see 3.4)

21 Miscellaneous Conditions

21.1 CIGUATERA FISH POISONING

West J Med 1995;163:31

Cause: Bioconcentration of heat-stable neurotoxins produced by marine dinoflagellates

Epidem: Worldwide; especially tropical Caribbean, subtropical N Atlantic; Pacific; in Miami, incidence of 5/100,000 population; from ingestion of reef fish such as grouper, red snapper, barracuda, amberjack; causes up to 10% of food poisonings in the U.S. (Arch Intern Med 1989;149:1735)

Risk for travelers: Significant in some areas, particularly w ingestion of larger fish or viscera

Incubation period: 6–24 hr

Sx: Watery diarrhea (30–90%), nausea/vomiting (30–70%), abd pain (30%), arthralgias, temperature reversal (30–80%), limb paresthesias (60–90%); circumoral paresthesias (30–90%)

Si: Bradycardia (10–30%), hypotension (10%)

Crs: GI sx resolve in 24 hr; neuro sx may last wk to mo

Rx: None

Prevent: Select smaller fish; avoid roe/viscera; do not eat barracuda

21.2 DELUSIONAL PARASITOSIS (OR PSYCHOGENIC PARASITOSIS)

CID 1998;26:924; Psychosomatics 1998;39:491

Cause: Fixed delusion of parasite infestation or infection, or persistent belief of same

Epidem: Unknown, but presumably more common in developed countries

Risk for travelers: Awareness of parasite exposure might contribute to its development in a predisposed individual, but most cases do not have an exotic travel hx

Sx: Often pruritus, anxiety, obsession w idea of infection to the degree it interferes w function

Si: Excoriated skin from scratches; "ziploc" sign noted by some (ie, pt often brings evidence of suspected cause in plastic bag, vial, etc. to office visit)

Crs: Can be persistent for yrs and quite debilitating

Rx: Success has been reported w pimozide (2–6 mg/d) and w risperidone (1–4 mg/d); check ECG before use, as pimozide incr Q-T interval; start w 1 mg/d; others recommend Haldol or other neuroleptic agents

21.3 PARALYTIC SHELLFISH POISONING

Cause: Bivalve mollusks w dinoflagellate *Gonylaux* sp ("red tides") that produce saxitoxin

Epidem: Worldwide; temperate coasts

Risk for travelers: Small, but incr in areas where shellfish flats not monitored

Incubation period: 30 min

Sx: Limb/circumoral paresthesias; "floating sensation," unsteadiness, vertigo; nausea

Si: cranial nerve palsies, ataxia

Crs: Up to 5% fatal due to respiratory failure w/in 1–12 h

Rx: supportive

Prevent: Avoid shellfish where safety cannot be assured (see also neurotoxin poisoning due to mussels w demoic acid (Nejm 1990;322:1781)

21.4 TROPICAL SPRUE

Cause: Unknown; prob bacterial (responds to antibiotics, household spread has been reported)
Epidem: Rare; most often dx in long-term travelers or immigrants; most cases in U.S. acquired in Haiti, Puerto Rico, India
Risk for travelers: Rare
Incubation period: mos to yrs
Sx: Diarrhea, weight loss, fatty stools
Si: Malabsorption
Crs: progressive sx until rx
Dx: Small bowel bx shows villus flattening
Rx: mos of antibiotics (usually tetracycline plus metronidazole, others)

Appendix 1

Geographic Distribution of Potential Health Hazards to Travelers

This section* is intended to give a *broad* indication of the health risks to which travelers may be exposed in various areas of the world and which they may not encounter in their usual place of residence.

In practice, to identify areas accurately and define the degree of risk likely in each of them is extremely difficult, if not impossible. For example, viral hepatitis A is ubiquitous, but the risk of infection varies not only according to area but also according to eating habits; hence, there may be more risk from communal eating in an area of low incidence than from eating in a private home in an area of high incidence. Generalizations may therefore be misleading. Current efforts to eradicate poliomyelitis worldwide are significantly reducing the risk of infection with wild poliovirus in almost all endemic areas.

Another factor is that tourism is an important source of income for many countries and to label specific areas as being of high risk for a disease may be misinterpreted. However, this does not absolve national health administrations from their responsibility to provide an accurate picture of the risks from communicable diseases that may be encountered in various parts of their countries.

* Reproduced from International Travel and Health (WHO, 1999) and Health Information for International Travel (CDC.)

AFRICA

Northern Africa (Algeria, Egypt, Libyan Arab Jamahiriya, Morocco, and Tunisia) is characterized by a generally fertile coastal area and a desert hinterland with oases that are often foci of infections.

Arthropod-borne diseases are unlikely to be a major problem to the traveler, although dengue fever, filariasis (focally in the Nile Delta), leishmaniasis, malaria, relapsing fever, Rift Valley fever, sandfly fever, typhus, and West Nile fever do occur in some areas.

Foodborne and waterborne diseases are endemic; the dysenteries and other diarrheal diseases are particularly common. Hepatitis A occurs throughout the area, and hepatitis E is endemic in some regions. Typhoid fever is common in some areas. Schistosomiasis (bilharziasis) is prevalent both in the Nile Delta area in Egypt and in the Nile valley; it occurs focally elsewhere in the area. Alimentary helminthic infections, brucellosis, and giardiasis are common. Echinococcosis (hydatid disease) may occur. Sporadic cases of cholera occur.

Other hazards. Poliomyelitis eradication efforts in northern Africa have been very successful and wild virus transmision in most of the area may have been interrupted. Egypt is the only country where confirmed cases of poliomyelitis were still reported in 1997. Trachoma, rabies, snakes, and scorpions are hazards in certain areas.

Sub-Saharan Africa (Angola, Benin, Burkina Faso, Burundi, Cameroon, Cape Verde, Central African Republic, Chad, Comoros, Congo, Côte d'Ivoire, Democratic Republic of Congo (formerly Zaire), Djibouti, Equatorial Guinea, Eritrea, Ethiopia, Gabon, Gambia, Ghana, Guinea, Guinea-Bissau, Kenya, Liberia, Madagascar, Malawi, Mali, Mauritania, Mauritius, Mozambique, Niger, Nigeria, Réunion, Rwanda, São Tomé and Principe, Senegal, Seychelles, Sierra Leone, Somalia, Sudan, Togo, Uganda, United Republic of Tanzania, Zambia, and Zimbabwe). In this area, entirely within the tropics, the vegetation varies from the tropical rain forests of the west and center to the wooded steppes of the east, and from the desert of the north through the Sahel and Sudan savannahs to the moist orchard savannah and woodlands north and south of the equator.

Many of the diseases listed below occur in localized rural foci and are confined to rural areas. They are mentioned so that the international traveler and the medical practitioner concerned may be aware of the diseases that may occur.

Arthropod-borne diseases are a major cause of morbidity. Malaria in the severe *Plasmodium falciparum* (malignant) form occurs throughout the area, except at over 2,600 meters altitude and in the islands of Réunion, and Seychelles. Various forms of filariasis are widespread; endemic foci of onchocerciasis (river blindness) exist in all the countries listed except in the greater part of Kenya and in Djibouti, Gambia, Mauritania, Mozambique, Somalia, Zambia, Zimbabwe, and the island countries of the Atlantic and Indian Oceans. However, onchocerciasis exists in the island of Bioko, Equatorial Guinea. Both cutaneous and visceral leishmaniasis may be found, particularly in the drier areas. Visceral leishmaniasis is epidemic in eastern and southern Sudan. Human trypanosomiasis (sleeping sickness), mainly in discrete foci, is reported from all countries except Djibouti, Eritrea, Gambia, Mauritania, Niger, Somalia, and the island countries of the Atlantic and Indian Oceans. The transmission of human trypanosomiasis is high in northwestern Uganda and very high in northern Angola, the Democratic Republic of Congo (mostly Equateur and Bandundu) and southern Sudan, and there is significant risk of infection for travelers visiting or working in rural areas. Relapsing fever and louse-, flea-, and tickborne typhus occur. Natural foci of plague* have been reported from Angola, Democratic Republic of Congo, Kenya, Madagascar, Mozambique, Uganda, the United Republic of Tanzania, and Zimbabwe. Tungiasis is widespread. Many viral diseases, some presenting as severe hemorrhagic fevers, are transmitted by mosquitos, ticks, sandflies, etc., which are found throughout this region. Large outbreaks of yellow fever occur periodically in the unvaccinated population.

Foodborne and waterborne diseases are highly endemic. Schistosomiasis (bilharziasis) is present throughout the area except in Cape Verde, Comoros, Djibouti, Réunion, and the Seychelles. Alimentary helminthic infections, the dysenteries and diarrheal diseases, including giardiasis, typhoid fever, and hepatitis A and E are widespread. Cholera is actively transmitted in many countries in this area. Dracunculiasis (Guinea worm) infection occurs in isolated foci. Paragonimiasis (oriental lung fluke) has been reported from Cameroon,

---

* A natural focus of plague is a strictly delimited area where ecological conditions ensure the persistence of plague in wild rodents (and occasionally other animals) for long periods of time, and where epizootics and periods of quiescence may alternate.

Gabon, Liberia and most recently from Equatorial Guinea.
Echinococcosis (hydatid disease) is widespread in animal-breeding areas.

Other diseases. Hepatitis B is hyperendemic. Poliomyelitis (also a foodborne and water-borne disease) is probably endemic in most countries except in Cape Verde, Comoros, Mauritius, Réunion, and the Seychelles. Trachoma is widespread. Among other diseases, certain frequently fatal arenavirus haemorrhagic fevers have attained notoriety. Lassa fever has a virus reservoir in a commonly found multimammate rat. Studies have shown that an appreciable reservoir exists in some rural areas of West Africa; people visiting these areas should take particular care to avoid rat-contaminated food or food containers, but the extent of the disease should not be exaggerated. The Ebola and Marburg hemorrhagic fevers are present but reported only infrequently.

Epidemics of meningococcal meningitis may occur throughout tropical Africa, particularly in the savannah areas during the dry season.

Other hazards include rabies and snake bites.

Southern Africa (Botswana, Lesotho, Namibia, St. Helena, South Africa, and Swaziland) varies physically from the Namib and Kalahari deserts to fertile plateaus and plains and to the more temperate climate of the southern coast.

Arthropod-borne diseases such as Crimean-Congo hemorrhagic fever, malaria, plague, relapsing fever, Rift Valley fever, tick-bite fever, and typhus, mainly tickborne, have been reported from most of this area except St. Helena, but except for malaria in certain areas, they are not likely to be a major health problem for the traveler. Trypanosomiasis (sleeping sickness) may occur in Botswana and Namibia.

Foodborne and waterborne diseases are common in some areas, particularly amebiasis and typhoid fever. Hepatitis A occurs in this area. Schistosomiasis (bilharziasis) is endemic in Botswana, Namibia, South Africa, and Swaziland.

Other hazards. The southern African countries are on the verge of becoming poliomyelitisfree, and the risk of contracting poliovirus is now low. Hepatitis B is hyperendemic. Snakes [and rabies*] may be a hazard in some areas.

---

* Editor's note: CDC addition.

THE AMERICAS

North America (Bermuda, Canada, Greenland, St. Pierre and Miquelon, and the United States of America [with Hawaii]) extends from the Arctic to the subtropical cays of the southern United States.

In 1994, an international commission certified the eradication of endemic wild poliovirus from the Americas. Ongoing surveillance in formerly endemic Central and South American countries confirms that poliovirus transmission remains interrupted.

The incidence of communicable disease is such that they are unlikely to prove a hazard for international travelers greater than that found in their own country. There are, of course, health risks, but in general, the precautions required are minimal. Certain diseases occasionally occur, such as plague, rabies in wildlife, including bats, Rocky Mountain spotted fever, tularemia, and arthropod-borne encephalitis. Recently, rodent-borne hantavirus has been identified, predominantly in the western states of the United States. Lyme disease is endemic in the northeastern United States, Mid-Atlantic, and the upper Midwest and the southwestern provinces of Canada. Occasional cases have been reported from the Pacific Northwest. During recent years, the incidence of certain food-borne diseases, e.g., salmonellosis, has increased in some regions. Other hazards include poisonous snakes, poison ivy, and poison oak. In the north, a serious hazard is the very low temperature in the winter.

In the United States, proof of immunization against diphtheria, measles, poliomyelitis, and rubella is now universally required for entry into school. In addition, the school entry requirements of most states include immunization against tetanus (49 states), pertussis (44 states), mumps (43 states), and hepatitis B (26 states).

Mainland Middle America (Belize, Costa Rica, El Salvador, Guatemala, Honduras, Mexico, Nicaragua, and Panama) ranges from the deserts of the north to the tropical rain forests of the southeast.

Of the *arthropod-borne diseases*, malaria and cutaneous and mucocutaneous leishmaniasis occur in all eight countries. Visceral leishmaniasis occurs in El Salvador, Guatemala, Honduras, Mexico, and Nicaragua. Onchocerciasis (river blindness) is found in two small foci in the south of Mexico and four dispersed foci in Guatemala. American trypanosomiasis (Chagas disease) has been reported to occur in localized foci in rural areas in all eight countries. Bancroftian filariasis is present in Costa Rica. Dengue fever and Venezuelan equine encephalitis may occur in all countries.

The *foodborne and waterborne diseases*, including amebic and bacillary dysenteries and other diarrheal diseases, and typhoid fever are very common throughout the area. All countries except Panama reported cases of cholera in 1996. Hepatitis A occurs throughout the area, and hepatitis E has been reported in Mexico. Helminthic infections are common. Paragonimiasis (oriental lung fluke) has been reported in Costa Rica, Honduras and Panama. Brucellosis occurs in the northern part of the area. Many *Salmonella typhi* infections from Mexico and *Shigella dysenteriae* type 1 infections from mainland Middle America as a whole have been caused by drug-resistant enterobacteria.

Other diseases. Rabies in animals (usually dogs and bats) is widespread throughout the area. Snakes may be a hazard in some areas.

Caribbean Middle America (Antigua and Barbuda, Aruba, Bahamas, Barbados, British Virgin Islands, Cayman Islands, Cuba, Dominica, Dominican Republic, Grenada, Guadeloupe, Haiti, Jamaica, Martinique, Montserrat, Netherlands Antilles, Puerto Rico, St. Christopher and Nevis, Saint Lucia, Saint Vincent and the Grenadines, Trinidad and Tobago, Turks and Caicos Islands, and the Virgin Islands [USA]). The islands, a number of them mountainous with peaks 1000–2500 m high, have an equable tropical climate with heavy rainstorms and high winds at certain times of the year.

Of the *arthropod-borne diseases*, malaria occurs in endemic form only in Haiti and in parts of the Dominican Republic. Diffuse cutaneous leishmaniasis was recently discovered in the Dominican Republic. Bancroftian filariasis occurs in Haiti and some other islands, and other filariases may occasionally be found. Human fascioliasis due to *Fasciola hepatica* is endemic in Cuba. Outbreaks of dengue fever occur in the area, and dengue hemorrhagic fever has also occurred. Tularemia has been reported from Haiti.

Of the *foodborne and waterborne diseases*, bacillary and amebic dysenteries are common, and hepatitis A is reported, particularly in the northern islands. No cases of cholera have been reported in the Caribbean. Schistosomiasis (bilharziasis) is endemic in the Dominican Republic, Guadeloupe, Martinique, Puerto Rico, and Saint Lucia, in each of which control operations are in progress. It may also occur sporadically in other islands.

Other diseases. Other hazards may occur from spiny sea urchins and coelenterates (coral and jellyfish) and snakes. Animal rabies, particularly in the mongoose, is reported from several islands.

Tropical South America (Bolivia, Brazil, Colombia, Ecuador, French Guiana, Guyana, Paraguay, Peru, Suriname, and Venezuela) covers the narrow coastal strip on the Pacific Ocean, the high Andean range with numerous peaks 5000–7000 m high, and the tropical rain forests of the Amazon basin, bordered to the north and south by savannah zones and dry tropical forest or scrub.

Arthropod-borne diseases are an important cause of ill health in rural areas. Malaria (in the *falciparum, malariae,* and *vivax* forms) occurs in all ten countries or areas, as do American trypanosomiasis (Chagas disease), and cutaneous and mucocutaneous leishmaniasis. There has been an increase of the latter in Brazil and Paraguay. Visceral leishmaniasis is endemic in northeast Brazil, with foci in other parts of Brazil, less frequent in Colombia and Venezuela, rare in Bolivia and Paraguay, and unknown in Peru. Endemic onchocerciasis occurs in isolated foci in rural areas in Ecuador, Venezuela, and northern Brazil. The bites of blackflies may cause unpleasant reactions. Bancroftian filariasis is endemic in parts of Brazil, Guyana and Suriname. Plague has been reported in natural foci in Bolivia, Brazil, Ecuador, and Peru. Among the arthropod-borne viral diseases, jungle yellow fever may be found in forest areas in all countries except Paraguay and areas east of the Andes; in Brazil it is confined to the northern and western states. Epidemics of viral encephalitis and dengue fever occur in some countries of this area. Bartonellosis, or Oroya fever, a sandfly-borne disease, occurs in arid river valleys on the western slopes of the Andes up to 3000 meters. Louse-borne typhus is often found in mountain areas of Colombia and Peru.

Foodborne and waterborne diseases are common and include amebiasis, diarrheal diseases, helminthic infections, and hepatitis A. The intestinal form of schistosomiasis (bilharziasis) is found in Brazil, Suriname, and north-central Venezuela. Paragonimiasis (oriental lung fluke) has been reported from Ecuador, Peru and Venezuela. Brucellosis is common and echinococcosis (hydatid disease) occurs, particularly in Peru. Bolivia, Brazil, Colombia, Ecuador, Peru, and Venezuela all reported autochthonous cases of cholera in 1996.

Other diseases include rodent-borne arenavirus hemorrhagic fever in Bolivia. Hepatitis B and D (delta hepatitis) are highly endemic in the Amazon Basin. Rabies has been reported from many of the countries in this area. Meningococcal meningitis occurs in epidemic outbreaks in Brazil.

Snakes and leeches may be a hazard in some areas.

Temperate South America (Argentina, Chile, Falkland Islands [Malvinas], and Uruguay). The mainland ranges from the Mediterranean climatic area of the western coastal strip over the Andes divide on to the steppes and desert of Patagonia in the south and to the prairies of the northeast.

The *arthropod-borne diseases* are relatively unimportant except for the occurrence of American trypanosomiasis (Chagas disease). Outbreaks of malaria occur in northwestern Argentina, and cutaneous leishmaniasis is also reported from the northeastern part of the country.

Of the *foodborne and waterborne diseases*, gastroenteritis (mainly salmonellosis) is relatively common in Argentina, especially in suburban areas and among children < 5 years of age. Some cases of cholera were reported in Argentina in 1996. Typhoid fever is not very common in Argentina but hepatitis A and intestinal parasitosis are widespread, the latter especially in the coastal region. Taeniasis (tapeworm), typhoid fever, viral hepatitis, and echinococcosis (hydatid disease) are reported from the other countries.

Other diseases. Anthrax is an occupational hazard in the three mainland countries. [Animal rabies is endemic in Argentina and Chile.*] Meningococcal meningitis occurs in the form of epidemic outbreaks in Chile. Rodent-borne hantavirus pulmonary syndrome has been identified in the north-central and southwestern regions of Argentina and in Chile.

ASIA

East Asia (China [including Hong Kong Special Administration Region], the Democratic People's Republic of Korea, Japan, Macao, Mongolia, and the Republic of Korea). The area includes the high mountain complexes, the desert and the steppes of the west, the various forest zones of the east, down to the subtropical forests of the southeast.

Among the *arthropod-borne diseases*, malaria now occurs in China, and in recent years cases have also been reported from the Korean peninsula. Although reduced in distribution and prevalence, bancroftian

---

* Editor's note: CDC addition.

and brugian filariasis are still reported in southern China. A resurgence of visceral leishmaniasis is occurring in China, and cutaneous leishmaniasis has been recently reported from Xinjiang, Uygur Autonomous Region. Plague may be found in China and Mongolia. Hemorrhagic fever with renal syndrome—rodent-borne, Korean hemorrhagic fever—is endemic except in Mongolia, and epidemics of dengue fever and Japanese encephalitis may occur in some areas. Mite-borne or scrub typhus may be found in scrub areas in southern China, certain river valleys in Japan, and in the Republic of Korea.

Foodborne and waterborne diseases such as diarrheal diseases and hepatitis A are common in most countries. Hepatitis E is prevalent in western China. The present endemic area of schistosomiasis (bilharziasis) is in the central Chang Jiang (Yangtze) river basin in China; active foci no longer occur in Japan. Clonorchiasis (oriental liver fluke) and paragonimiasis (oriental lung fluke) are reported in China, Japan, Macao and the Republic of Korea, and fasciolopsiasis (giant intestinal fluke) in China. Brucellosis occurs in China. Cholera may occur in some countries in this area.

Other diseases. Hepatitis B is highly endemic. Low levels of poliomyelitis morbidity are reported from China and Mongolia. Trachoma and leptospirosis occur in China. Outbreaks of meningococcal meningitis occur in Mongolia. [Rabies is endemic in China and Korea.*] Poliomyelitis eradication activities have rapidly reduced poliovirus transmission.

Eastern South Asia (Brunei Darussalam, Cambodia, Indonesia, Lao People's Democratic Republic, Malaysia, Myanmar [Burma], the Philippines, Singapore, Thailand, and Vietnam). From the tropical rain and monsoon forests of the northwest, the area extends through the savannah and the dry tropical forests of the Indochina peninsula, returning to the tropical rain and monsoon forests of the islands bordering the South China Sea.

The *arthropod-borne diseases* are an important cause of morbidity throughout the area. Malaria and filariasis are endemic in many parts of the rural areas of all the countries or areas—except for malaria in Brunei Darussalam and Singapore, where normally only imported cases occur. Plague exists in Myanmar and Vietnam. Japanese encephalitis, dengue and dengue hemorrhagic fever can occur in epidemics in both urban and

---

* Editor's note: CDC addition.

rural areas. Mite-borne typhus has been reported in deforested areas in most countries.

Foodborne and waterborne diseases are common. Cholera and other watery diarrheas, amebic and bacillary dysentery, typhoid fever, and hepatitis A and E may occur in all countries in the area. Schistosomiasis (bilharziasis) is endemic in the Southern Philippines and in central Sulawesi (Indonesia) and occurs in small foci in the Mekong Delta in Vietnam. Among helminthic infections, fasciolopsiasis (giant intestinal fluke) may be acquired in most countries in the area; clonorchiasis (oriental liver fluke) in the Indochina peninsula; opisthorchiasis (cat liver fluke) in the Indochina peninsula, the Philippines, and Thailand; and paragonimiasis in most countries. Melioidosis can occur sporadically throughout the area.

Other diseases. Hepatitis B is highly endemic. The only remaining focus of poliovirus transmission is in the Mekong Delta area of Cambodia and southern Vietnam. Poliovirus transmission has probably been interrupted in Indonesia, Lao People's Democratic Republic, Malaysia, Myanmar, the Philippines, and Thailand. Trachoma exists in Indonesia, Myanmar, Thailand, and Vietnam.

Other hazards include rabies, snake bites, and leeches.

Middle South Asia (Afghanistan, Armenia, Azerbaijan, Bangladesh, Bhutan, Georgia, India, Islamic Republic of Iran, Kazakhstan, Kyrgyzstan, Maldives, Nepal, Pakistan, Sri Lanka, Tajikistan, Turkmenistan, and Uzbekistan). Bordered for the most part by high mountain ranges in the north, the area extends from steppes and desert in the west to monsoon and tropical rain forests in the east and south.

Arthropod-borne diseases are endemic in all these countries except for malaria in Georgia, Kazakhstan, Krygyzstan, the Maldives, Turkmenistan and Uzbekistan. There are small foci of malaria in Armenia, Azerbaijan, and Tajikistan. In some of the other countries, malaria occurs in urban as well as rural areas. Filariasis is common in Bangladesh, India, and the southwestern coastal belt of Sri Lanka. Sand fly fever is on the increase. A sharp rise in the incidence of visceral leishmaniasis has been observed in Bangladesh, India and Nepal. In Pakistan, it is mainly reported from the north (Baltisan). Cutaneous leishmaniasis occurs in Afghanistan, India (Rajasthan), the Islamic Republic of Iran, and Pakistan. There are very small foci of cutaneous and visceral leishmaniasis in Azerbaijan and Tajikistan. There is evidence that natural foci of plague exist in India and Kazakhstan. Tickborne relapsing fever is reported from Afghanistan, India, and the Islamic

Republic of Iran, and typhus occurs in Afghanistan and India. Outbreaks of dengue fever may occur in Bangladesh, India, Pakistan, and Sri Lanka, and the hemorrhagic form has been reported from eastern India and Sri Lanka. Japanese encephalitis has been reported from the eastern part of the area and Crimean-Congo hemorrhagic fever from the western part. Another tickborne hemorrhagic fever has been reported in forest areas of Karnataka State in India and in a rural area of Rawalpindi District in Pakistan.

Foodborne and waterborne diseases are common throughout the area, in particular cholera and other watery diarrheas, the dysenteries, typhoid fever, hepatitis A and E, and helminthic infections. Large epidemics of hepatitis E can occur. Giardiasis is common in the area. A very limited focus of urinary schistosomiasis (bilharziasis) persists in the southwest of the Islamic Republic of Iran. Brucellosis and echinococcosis (hydatid disease) are found in many countries in the area.

Other diseases. Hepatitis B is endemic. Outbreaks of meningococcal meningitis have been reported in India and Nepal. Poliomyelitis eradication activities have begun in all countries in the area, rapidly reducing the risk of infection with wild poliovirus. However, surveillance data are incomplete and poliovirus transmission should still be assumed to be a risk to travelers in most countries, especially in the Indian subcontinent. Trachoma is common in Afghanistan, in parts of India, the Islamic Republic of Iran, Nepal, and Pakistan. Snakes and the presence of rabies in animals are hazards in most of the countries in the area.

Western South Asia (Bahrain, Cyprus, Iraq, Israel, Jordan, Kuwait, Lebanon, Oman, Qatar, Saudi Arabia, Syrian Arab Republic, Turkey, the United Arab Emirates, and Yemen). The area ranges from the mountains and steppes of the northwest to the large deserts and dry tropical scrub of the south.

The *arthropod-borne diseases*, except for malaria in certain areas, are not a major hazard for the traveler. Malaria does not exist in Kuwait and no longer occurs in Bahrain, Cyprus, Israel, Jordan, Lebanon, or Qatar. Its incidence in Oman, the Syrian Arab Republic, and the United Arab Emirates is low, but elsewhere it is endemic in certain rural areas. Cutaneous leishmaniasis is reported throughout the area; visceral leishmaniasis, although rare throughout most of the area, is common in central Iraq, in the southwest of Saudi Arabia, in the northwest of the Syrian Arab Republic, in Turkey (southeast Anatolia only) and in the west of Yemen. Murine and tickborne typhus can occur in certain countries. Tickborne relapsing fever may occur. Crimean-Congo hemorrhagic fever has been reported from Iraq. Limited foci of onchocerciasis are reported in Yemen.

The *foodborne and waterborne diseases* are a major hazard in most countries. The typhoid fevers and hepatitis A exist in all countries. Schistosomiasis (bilharziasis) occurs in Iraq, Saudi Arabia, the Syrian Arab Republic, and Yemen. Dracunculiasis (guinea worm) occurs in isolated foci in Yemen. Taeniasis (tapeworm) is reported from many of the countries. Brucellosis is reported from most countries, and there are foci of echinococcosis (hydatid disease).

Other diseases. Hepatitis B is endemic. The risk of poliomyelitis (also a food-borne and water-borne disease) is low in most countries of the area, with the exception of Yemen. Trachoma and animal rabies are found in many countries in the area.

The greatest hazards to pilgrims to Mecca and Medina are heat and water depletion if the period of the Hajj coincides with the hot season.

EUROPE

Northern Europe (Belarus, Belgium, Czech Republic, Denmark [with the Faroe Islands], Estonia, Finland, Germany, Iceland, Ireland, Latvia, Lithuania, Luxembourg, Netherlands, Norway, Poland, Republic of Moldova, Russian Federation, Slovakia, Sweden, Ukraine, and the United Kingdom [with the Channel Islands and the Isle of Man]. The area encompassed by these countries extends from the broadleaf forests and the plains of the west to the boreal and mixed forest to be found as far east as the Pacific Ocean.

The incidence of communicable diseases in most countries is such that they are unlikely to prove a hazard to international travelers greater than that found in their own country. There are, of course, health risks, but in most areas very few precautions are required.

Of the *arthropod-borne diseases*, there are very small foci of tickborne typhus in east and central Siberia. Tickborne encephalitis, for which a vaccine exists, and Lyme disease may occur throughout forested areas where vector ticks are found. Rodent-borne hemorrhaghic fever with renal syndrome is now recognized as occurring at low endemic levels in this area.

The *foodborne and waterborne diseases* reported, other than the ubiquitous diarrheal diseases are taeniasis (tapeworm) and trichinellosis in parts of northern Europe, diphyllobothriasis (fish tapeworm) from the freshwater fish around the Baltic Sea area. *Fasciola hepatica* infection can occur. Hepatitis A occurs in the eastern European countries. The incidence of certain food-borne diseases, e.g., salmonellosis and campylobacteriosis, is increasing significantly in some of these countries.

Other diseases. All endemic countries in the area are now making intense efforts to eradicate poliomyelitis. Rabies is endemic in wild animals (particularly foxes) in rural areas of northern Europe. In recent years, Belarus, the Russian Federation, and Ukraine have experienced extensive epidemics of diphtheria. Diphtheria cases, mostly imported from these three countries, have also been reported from neighboring countries: Estonia, Finland, Latvia, Lithuania, Poland, and the Republic of Moldova.

A climatic hazard in part of northern Europe is the extreme cold in winter.

Southern Europe (Albania, Andorra, Austria, Bosnia and Herzegovina, Bulgaria, Croatia, France, Gibraltar, Greece, Hungary, Italy, Liechtenstein, Malta, Monaco, Portugal [with the Azores and Madeira], Romania, San Marino, Slovenia, Spain [with the Canary Islands], Switzerland, and the Former Yugoslav Republic of Macedonia, and Yugoslavia. The area extends from the broadleaf forests in the northwest and the mountains of the Alps to the prairies and, in the south and southeast, the scrub vegetation of the Mediterranean.

Among the *arthropod-borne diseases*, sporadic cases of murine and tickborne typhus and mosquito-borne West Nile fever occur in some countries bordering the Mediterranean littoral. Both cutaneous and visceral leishmaniasis and sandfly fever are also reported from this area. Recently an increasing number of *Leishmania*/HIV co-infections have been notified from France, Greece, Italy, Portugal and Spain. Tickborne encephalitis, for which a vaccine exists, Lyme disease, and rodent-borne hemorrhagic fever with renal syndrome may occur in the eastern and southern parts of the area.

The *foodborne and waterborne diseases*—bacillary dysentery and other diarrheas, and typhoid fever—are more common in the summer and autumn months, with a high incidence in the southeastern and southwestern parts of the area. Brucellosis can occur in the extreme southwest and southeast and echinococcosis (hydatid disease) in the southeast. Fasciola hepatica infection has been reported from different countries in the area. The incidence of certain foodborne diseases, e.g., salmonellosis and campylobacteriosis, is increasing significantly in some of these countries.

Other diseases. All countries in southern Europe where poliomyelitis was until recently endemic are conducting eradication activities, and the risk of infection in most countries is very low. However, a large poliomyelitis outbreak occurred in 1996 in Albania, also affecting Greece and Yugoslavia; it had been interrupted by the end of 1996. Hepatitis B is endemic in the southern part of eastern Europe (Albania, Bulgaria, and Romania). Rabies in animals* exists in most countries of southern Europe except Albania, Gibraltar, Greece, Italy, Malta, Monaco, the former Yugoslav Republic of Macedonia, Portugal, and Spain, except Ceuta/Melilla.

OCEANIA

Australia, New Zealand, and the Antarctic. In Australia the mainland has tropical monsoon forests in the north and east, dry tropical forests, savannah and deserts in the center, and Mediterranean scrub and subtropical forests in the south. New Zealand has a temperate climate with the North Island characterized by subtropical forests and the South Island by steppe vegetation and hardwood forests.

International travelers to Australia and New Zealand will, in general, not be subjected to the hazards of communicable diseases to an extent greater than that found in their own country.

Arthropod-borne diseases (mosquito-borne epidemic polyarthritis and viral encephalitis) may occur in some rural areas of Australia. Occasional outbreaks of dengue have occurred in northern Australia in recent years.

Other hazards. Coelenterates (corals and jellyfish) may prove a hazard to the sea-bather, and heat is a hazard in the northern and central parts of Australia. Insectivorous and fruit-eating bats in Australia have been found to harbor a virus related to rabies virus and therefore should be avoided.

Melanesia and Micronesia-Polynesia (American Samoa, Cook Islands, Easter Island, Federated States of Micronesia, Fiji, French

* Editor's note: CDC addition.

Polynesia, Guam, Kiribati, Marshall Islands, Nauru, New Caledonia, Niue, Palau, Papua New Guinea, Pitcairn, Samoa, Solomon Islands, Tokelau, Tonga, Trust Territory of the Pacific Islands, Tuvalu, Vanuatu, Wake Island [U.S.] and the Wallis and Futuna Islands). The area covers an enormous expanse of ocean with the larger, mountainous, tropical and monsoon rainforest-covered islands of the west giving way to the smaller, originally volcanic peaks and coral islands of the east.

Arthropod-borne diseases occur in the majority of the islands. Malaria is endemic in Papua New Guinea, Solomon Islands and Vanuatu. Filariasis is widespread but its prevalence varies. Mite-borne typhus has been reported from Papua New Guinea. Dengue fever, including its hemorrhagic form, can occur in epidemics in most islands.

Foodborne and waterborne diseases such as the diarrheal diseases, typhoid fever and helminthic infections are commonly reported. Biointoxication may occur from raw or cooked fish and shellfish. Hepatitis A occurs in this area.

Other diseases. Hepatitis B is endemic. No cases of poliomyelitis have been reported from any of these islands for more than 5 years. Trachoma occurs in parts of Melanesia.

Hazards to bathers are coelenterates, poisonous fish, and sea snakes.

Appendix 2

Antiparasitic Drugs

- Albendazole (Zentel); for cutaneous and visceral larval migrans, pinworms, hookworm, hydatid cysts and cysticercosis, whipworm; adverse effects: occasionally reversible alopecia, LFT elevations, abdominal pain; rarely leukopenia, alopecia, elevated LFTs
- Artemether (Nejm 1996;335:69, 76, 124) 2–4 mg/kg im qd for cerebral falcip malaria; adv effects: long QT syndrome
- Atovaquone (Mepron) 750 mg po tid × 21 d for pneumocystis, adverse effects: rash, nausea, diarrhea
Atovaquone/proguanil (Malarone) 250 mg/100 mg combination tablet for prophylaxis (one tab qd and 7 d after return) and treatment (4 tabs/d × 3d=adult Rx) of malaria.
- Bithionol (Bitin) 30–50 mg/kg po × 10–15 doses for lung fluke and *Fasciola hepatica*; available from CDC only; adverse effects: photosensitivity, emesis, diarrhea, urticaria; rarely leukopenia, hepatitis
- Chloroquine HCl, chloroquine phosphate (Aralen) 600 mg base (1 gm) or 10 mg/kg, then 300 mg base (500 mg) or 5 mg/kg at 6, 24, and 48 h for malaria; 300 mg or 5 mg/kg base po q 1 wk for prophylaxis; also used occasionally in amebiasis; adverse effects: emesis, headache/confusion, pruritus, alopecia, weight loss, worse preexisting dermatitis, myalgias; rarely irreversible retinal damage, nail changes, neuronal deafness, peripheral neuropathy, myopathy, heart block, hematemesis
- Crotamiton (Eurax) 10% soln topically for scabies; adverse effects: rash, conjunctivitis
- Dapsone (DDS, diaminodiphenylsulfone) 100 mg po qd to prevent *P. carinii* pneumonia (Ann IM 1995;123:584); adverse effects: rashes, headache, gi, mono syndrome, etc.

- Dehydroemetine 1–1.5 mg/kg/d im up to 5 d for severe amebiasis; adverse effects: arrhythmias, muscle weakness; occasional diarrhea, emesis, peripheral neuropathy, CHF, headache
- Diethylcarbamazine (Hetrazan) 50 mg or 1 mg/kg po on day 1, 50 mg or 1 mg/kg po tid day 2, 100 mg or 2 mg/kg po tid day 3, then 9 mg/kg/d divided for 21 d crs for filariasis; adverse effects: allergic/febrile reactions w heavy microfilarial load, gi sx; rarely encephalopathy
- Diethylmethylbenzamide (DEET) (Ann IM 1998;128:934) 35% slow release (HourGuard), or 6.5–10% SR formulations; insect repellant, lasts 3–4 hr, better than Skin-So-Soft, Citronella, or others
- Eflornithine (difluoromethylornithine, DFMO, Ornidyl) for trypanosomiasis; adverse effects: anemia, leukopenia, diarrhea, thrombocytopenia, seizures; rarely deafness
- Furazolidone (Furoxone) 100 mg or 1.5 mg/kg po qid × 7–10 d for giardiasis; adverse effects: nausea/vomiting, anaphylactoid reactions, hypoglycemia, headache; rarely hemolytic anemia if G6PD-deficient, Antabuse reaction w alcohol, polyneuritis
- Iodoquinol (Yodoxin) 650 mg or 10–12 mg/kg po tid × 20 d for amebiasis and *Dientamoeba fragilis*; adverse effects: rash, acne, thyroidomegaly, diarrhea, anal itching; rarely optic neuritis; optic atrophy, peripheral neuropathy
- Ivermectin (Mectizan) for onchocercal filariasis; adverse effects: malaise/fever w heavy worm load
- Lindane (Kwell) topically for lice and scabies; adverse effects: rash, headache, conjunctivitis; rarely seizures, aplastic anemia; all increased if skin vasodilated, eg, in warm weather
- Malathion (Ovide) 0.5% topically for lice; adverse effects: local skin irritation
- Mebendazole (Vermox) varying doses for pinworm, filariasis, hookworm, whipworm, visceral larval migrans, ascariasis; adverse effects: diarrhea, abdominal pain; rarely leukopenia, hypospermia
- Mefloquine (Lariam) 250 mg or 25 mg/kg × 1; adverse effects: vertigo, gi sx, nightmares, headache, confusion; rarely psychoses, seizures, shock, coma, paresthesias
- Melarsoprol (Arsobal) 2–3.6 mg/kg/d iv × 3 d 1st week, then 3.6 mg/kg/d × 3 d iv 2nd and 3rd wk for CNS trypanosomiasis/Chagas' disease; adverse effects: cardiac injury, albuminuria,

hypertension, colic, Herxheimer reaction, encephalopathy, emesis, peripheral neuropathy

- Metronidazole (Flagyl) various doses for amebiasis, trichomonas, *Balantidium coli*, tapeworms, giardia, hookworm, whipworm, visceral larval migrans; adverse effects: nausea/vomiting, headache, metallic taste, insomnia, stomatitis, rash, dysuria, paresthesias, Antabuse reaction to alcohol; rarely seizures, colitis, encephalopathy, neuropathy, pancreatitis. No increase in cancer risk (Nejm 1979;301:519)
- Niclosamide (Niclocide) 50 mg/kg up to 2 gm × 1 chewed for fasciolopsis fluke and dwarf tapeworm; adverse effects: nausea, abdominal pain
- Nifurtimox (Lampit) 8–10 mg/kg/d po in qid doses × 120 d, double doses for children × 90 d for *T. cruzi* (Chagas' disease); adverse effects: anorexia, emesis, weight loss, sleep changes, tremor, paresthesias, polyneuritis, memory loss; rarely seizures, fever, pulmonary infiltrates
- Oxamniquine (Vansil) 15 mg/kg × 1, 10 mg/kg bid × 1 d for children, for *Schistosoma mansoni*; adverse effects: headache, fever, somnolence, diarrhea, rash, insomnia, LFT elevations, orange urine; rarely seizures, psych changes
- Paromomycin (aminosidine, Humatin) 25–30 mg/kg/d in tid dosing × 7 d for amebiasis, *Dientamoeba fragilis*, cryptosporidium; adverse effects: gi sx, VIII nerve damage (hearing), renal injury
- Pentamidine (Pentam) 2–4 mg/kg im/iv qd × 14–21 d for leishmaniasis, pneumocystis; adverse effects: hypotension, hypoglycemia/diabetes induction, emesis, renal damage, gi sx, local injection pain, hypocalcemia, cardiotoxicity, hepatotoxicity, delirium, rash; rarely anaphylaxis, pancreatitis, hyperkalemia because is similar to triamterene (Ann IM 1995;122:103)
- Permethrin (Nix, Elimite) topically 1% for lice, 5% for scabies; adverse effects: local irritation
- Praziquantel (Biltricide) 25 mg/kg tid × 1 d for flukes, schistosomiasis, tapeworms; adverse effects: malaise, sedation, fever, eosinophilia, abdominal pain; rarely rash
- Primaquine 15 mg base (6.3 mg)/d or 0.3 mg base/kg/d × 14 d, or 45 mg base/wk × 8 wk for prevention of *P. vivax* and *ovale* relapse after leave area; adverse effects: hemolytic anemia in G6PD pts, neutropenia, gi sx; rare CNS sx, hypertension, arrhythmias

- Pyrantel pamoate (Antiminth) 11 mg/kg (max = 1 gm) × 3 d for hookworm, 11 mg/kg × 1 repeat in 2 wk for pinworm; adverse effects: gi sx, headache, rash, fever
- Pyrethrins + Piperonyl butoxide (RID) topically for lice; adverse effects: allergic reaction
- Pyrimethamine (Daraprim) 25–100 mg (1 mg/kg)/d × 3–4 wk w sulfadiazine for toxoplasmosis; adverse effects: folate deficiency; rarely rash, emesis, seizures
- Pyrimethamine-sulfadoxine (Fansidar), 3 tabs × 1 on last day of quinine for resistant falcip malaria; adverse effects: folate deficiency; rarely fatal Steven-Johnson syndrome, emesis, seizures
- Quinacrine (Atabrine) 100 mg or 2 mg/kg tid × 5 d for giardiasis; no longer available in U.S.; adverse effects: headache, emesis, diarrhea, yellow skin, psychoses, insomnia, blue nails, rash like psoriasis
- Sodium stibogluconate (Pentostam) (pentavalent antimony) 20 mg Sb/kg/d iv/im × 21–28 d for leishmaniasis; adverse effects: myalgias, arthralgias (90%), LFT elevations (25%), T-wave inversions (30%), weakness, colic, bradycardia, leukopenia; rarely diarrhea, rash, MI, hemoytic anemia, renal damage
- Spiramycin (Rovamycine) 50–100 mg/kg up to 3–4 gm/d × 3–4 wk for toxoplasmosis during pregnancy; adverse effects: gi sx; rarely allergic reactions
- Suramin Na (Germanin) 100-mg test dose then 20 mg/kg up to 1 gm iv days 1, 3, 7, 14, 21 for sleeping sickness; adverse effects: emesis, urticaria, paresthesias, neuropathy, renal damage, optic atrophy
- Thiabendazole (Mintezol) various doses for angiostrongyliasis, cutaneous larval migrans, dracunculus, strongyloides; adverse effects: nausea/vomiting, vertigo, leukopenia, crystalluria, rash, hallucinations, erythema multiforme, smell changes; rarely tinnitus, cholestasis, seizures, angioneurotic edema

Appendix 3

Bibliography

BOOKS AND HANDBOOKS

Auerbach PS, ed. *Wilderness Medicine—Management of Wilderness and Environmental Emergencies*. 3rd ed. St. Louis: Mosby; 1995. (Comprehensive textbook—the key reference for wilderness medicine information.)

Auerbach PS, Donner HJ, Weiss EA. *Field Guide to Wilderness Medicine*. St. Louis: Mosby; 1999. (Good handbook for advice on most wilderness and environmental health ailments.)

CDC. *Health Information for International Travel, 1999–2000*. Atlanta: DHHS; 2001. (Excellent resource for physicians with up to date information for preparation of travelers: updated annually.) Available from Superintendent of Documents, Government Printing Office, Washington DC 2002; order #017-023-00202-3. (Call 202-512-1800)

Dupont H, Steffen R. *Textbook of Travel Medicine and Health*. Hamilton, Ontario: Decker Inc.; 2000. (Comprehensive resource for health care providers, travel clinics by two leading travel medicine experts.)

Guerrant R, Krogstad D, Maguire J, et al. *Tropical Infectious Diseases: Principles, Pathogens, & Practice*. New York: Churchill-Livingstone; 1999. (Detailed and authoritative multiauthored textbook by leading tropical medicine clinicians and researchers.)

Jong EC, McMullen R. *The Travel and Tropical Medicine Manual*. 2nd ed. Philadelphia: Saunders; 1998. (Highly regarded and comprehensive handbook.)

Mandell GL, Bennett JE, Dolin R. *Principles and Practice of Infectious Diseases*; 4th ed. New York: Churchill Livingstone; 2000. (Authoritative cornerstone for infectious disease physicians and others.)

Plotkin SA, Orenstein WA, eds. *Vaccines*. 3rd ed. Philadelphia: Saunders; 1999.

Rose SR. *International Travel Health Guide*. Northampton, MA: Travel Medicine Inc; 2000. (A superb manual for the inveterate traveler and health care professional.)

Steffen R, Dupont HL. *Manual of Travel Medicine and Health*. Hamilton, Ontario: Decker; 1999. (Comprehensive handbook of travel health with extensive epidemiologic information on disease risk and on vaccines.)

Thompson RF. *Travel & Routine Immunizations*. Milwaukee: Shoreland; 2000. (A detailed reference for office use that focuses on vaccines.)

Warren KS, Mahmoud AAF. *Tropical and Geographic Medicine*. New York: McGraw-Hill; 1984.

WHO. *International Travel and Health*. Geneva: Author. (Updated annually.)

Wilson ME. *A World Guide to Infections: Diseases, Diagnosis, Treatment*. Oxford: Oxford University Press; 1991. (The best resource on geographic risk of disease.)

PRIMARILY TARGETED FOR TRAVELERS

See Rose above (*International Travel Health Guide*).

Wolfe MS. *Health Hints for the Tropics*. American Society of Tropical Medicine; 1998. (Highly recommended.) Call ASTMH at 703-790-1745.

TRAVEL MEDICINE RESOURCES

NEWSLETTERS

Travel Medicine Advisor. Excellent source of travel health information with bimonthly updates. American Health Consultants, P.O. Box 740060, Atlanta, GA 30374.

Traveling Healthy. Editor Karl Neumann MD. Another excellent resource with regular updated reports.

WEBSITES: UPDATED GENERAL INFORMATION ON TRAVEL HEALTH

http://www.cdc.gov—Centers for Disease Control and Prevention. Includes text of latest Health Information for Travelers with recommendations for immunizations and malaria prevention, and updates on emerging health risks. (817-394-8747)

http://www.state.gov—U.S. State Department travel advisories, consular information, etc. (202-647-6575)

http://www.cdc.gov/nip—CDC National Immunization Program with information on vaccine use, adverse events, disease risk, etc.

http://www.hc-sc.gc.ca—Canadian Laboratory Centre for Disease Control. Canadian health advisory information; search under "travel."

http://www.who.org—World Health Organization. Check "International Travel and Health Information" page.

http://www.ch/wer/—WHO. Weekly epidemiologic reports.

http://www.cdc.gov/epo/mmwr/mmwr.htm—MMWR. (CDC-generated weekly epidemiologic reports.)

http://www.fas.org/promed—Reports of emerging disease issues and outbreaks. ProMED c/o Federation of American Scientists, 307 Massachusetts Ave, Washington, DC 20002.

WEBSITES: INFORMATION ON TRAVEL CLINICS, OTHER RESOURCES

http://www.astmh.org—American Society of Tropical Medicine and Hygiene. Maintains lists of travel clinics, other dependable resources.

http://www.istm.org—International Society of Travel Medicine. Also with lists of clinics, etc.

http://www.medicalert.org—Medical Alert Foundation.

http://www.asirt.org/about.cfm—Association for Safe International Road Travel. Lists road conditions, accident rates, etc. for many parts of the world.

http://www.diversalertnetwork—Divers Alert Network (DAN).

WEBSITES: FOR TRAVELERS:

http://www.travelmed.com—general information.

http://www.medicineplanet.com—general information.

http://www.tripprep.com—Shoreland Travel Health On-line.

International Association for Medical Assistance to Travelers:
   http:www.iamat.org OR
   http:www.sentex.netNIAMAT

Travax Pre Travel Advice:
   http:www.shoreland.com

Index

Page numbers followed by f, m, or t indicate figures, maps, or tables, respectively.